Letters of Commendations for

The United States Marshal Service and the entire Law Enforcement Community has a great friend in Instructor David Kahn. The Krav Maga System is a no-nonsense self-defense system that deals with threats at all levels ... I could not recommend a more qualified instructor.
—**Lori M. Bell**, U.S. Marshal, United States Marshal Service.

I had the awesome experience recently, along with several other Special Agents of the Detroit FBI, of participating in a Krav Maga session with David Kahn and Rick Blitstein. As a Defensive Tactics Instructor for the Detroit Field Division, I had skepticism about the program due to its reputation as a style too aggressive for the needs of law enforcement. I was soon shown otherwise. David Kahn and Rick Blitstein are well versed on the needs of the modern day law enforcement officer, and are attuned to issues related to liability, applicability, and simplicity. In fact, the entire concept of Krav Maga is based upon simplicity. Knowing most officers and departments are not in a position to train regularly or rigorously enough to master complicated systems, Dave and Rick have successfully adapted key techniques of weapon retention, weapon take-away, control techniques, and personal weapons. I believe most officers can come away with sufficient skill to apply these techniques in just a four-hour session. I was particularly impressed with the concept of "Retzev. ... It is quite different from standard defensive tactics currently being employed ... Rick and Dave have great enthusiasm and relate comfortably with law enforcement personnel because they have taken the time to know and understand their needs. They recognize the differences in physical abilities of officers. They understand that to be effective, the techniques must be user friendly and the skills must be sustainable without having to be drilled weekly. It is apparent that these factors were foremost in their minds when they set up our session. [They] ... have brought an already top notch fighting system to another level, a level all law enforcement should be pursuing for the safety of its officers and the citizens.
—**John E. Ouellet**, Special Agent, FBI, Detroit.

I would like to take this opportunity to thank you for opening your facility and sharing your expertise in Israeli Krav Maga with members of the New Jersey State Police, Executive Protection Unit. The simplicity of the moves, coupled with the effectiveness of the techniques, makes this training curriculum useful in real world situations. I particularly liked the disarming training and simultaneous 'block and strike' techniques utilized ... Israeli Krav Maga has further prepared the New Jersey State Police, Executive Protection Unit, in achieving our mission ...
—**Lt. Frank Maimone**, Training Officer, Executive Protection Unit, New Jersey State Police.

I would like to take this opportunity to thank you for providing your expert instruction during the Israeli Krav Maga Defensive Tactics Course hosted by the Firearms/Self-Defense Training

Unit, Training Bureau, at the NJSP Academy, Sea Girt, NJ. Israeli Krav Maga ... a cutting edge system geared to ending confrontations in an efficient manner while limiting collateral damage to the trooper and innocent bystanders. Again, I would like to thank you for providing this critical instruction to our troopers, and I know the Academy Staff is looking forward to working with you in the future...

—**(Col) Joseph Fuentes**, Superintendent, New Jersey State Police.

Your professionalism and motivation were most inspiring and clearly showed in all facets of training. Having attended various self-defense and weapons retention courses, I can say without reservation that the techniques you taught are superior to anything I have learned. ... The tactics learned are essential in officer survival and situational awareness and taught those trained how to detect a confrontation and avoid a worsening situation. I firmly believe that your system should be incorporated into Homeland Security training including our training plan and all officers taught the benefit of Israeli krav maga. Semper Paratus.

—**Officer Mark A. Hanafee**, Coast Guard Police, Training Officer.

I am writing this letter in reference to the outstanding training conducted by you .... at Fort Dix, New Jersey. The tactical training given was professional, thorough, and proved essential to officer safety. ... Your Krav Maga tactics were second to none and your level of instruction was intense. Semper Paratus.

—**Petty Officer Kevin A. Colon**, United States Coast Guard, Small Arms Instructor (HH).

"Thank you for taking time out of your busy schedule to come to the New Jersey State Police Academy and conduct a weapon retention seminar for our SWAT Team Troopers. The Krav Maga techniques that were taught were easily learned and very effective ... The proven techniques of Krav Maga provide any police officer with the most effective means possible to fend off an attacker and retain their weapon. . . Your knowledge, skill and personality create a great learning environment for even the most hardcore Troopers in the New Jersey State Police. ... We look forward to continuing our relationship with you and the Israeli Krav Maga Association.

—**Trooper I. Paul Miller 4476**, Division Firearms Coordinator, New Jersey State Police.

Critical to a law enforcement professional's survival are the will to survive and the skills to survive. We accept the reality that our lives can be permanently altered in moment. That is where the Israeli Krav Maga 'contact combat' system comes in and provides the skills to survive. When the need to deliver is paramount Israeli Krav Maga is truly an effective practical fighting system. Thank you for the amazing demonstration and hands on training you provided for the New

Jersey Women in Law Enforcement … The instruction provided by you, Abel Kahn, and Mike Delahanty was first class and the application to law enforcement professionals is endless. Our members are still talking about it! You and your instructors were the ultimate gentlemen and made every member feel included and engaged with your style and grace. The members of New Jersey Women in Law Enforcement look forward to a long relationship with you and your instructional staff.

> —**C. Lynn Cetonze**, President, New Jersey Women in Law Enforcement.

On behalf of the first class of the Mercer County Police Academy we would like to extend our deepest and most sincere gratitude for the training … We have been studying defensive tactics throughout our entire time at the academy, but nothing is as impressive or seemed as effective and the Israeli Krav Maga techniques you taught us. We have had some exposure to Israeli Krav Maga through some of our instructors, who are students at your school. The difference in seeing what this discipline can do by someone who has mastered it was beyond impressive. Your style of teaching was as impressive and just as effective as your craft: quick, meaningful, and to the point. You showed us exactly what we needed to do, and your vigilance while instructing allowed you to step in and quickly adjust and correct any problems we were experiencing. The opportunity to benefit from your instruction will be remembered as one of the most fortunate experiences in our academy. We feel these tactics can truly make the difference between life and death in a dangerous encounter.

> —**Mercer County Police Cadets**, Class 01–07.

I wanted to seize this opportunity to thank you for taking time out of your busy schedule to come to Stewart Air National Guard Base and train my Security Forces. Our new mission will require my people to operate and patrol outside the wire in hostile and dangerous environments and the training and techniques you taught them may someday save their lives or the lives of their fellow Wingmen. We have incorporated the techniques you shared with us into our own training and we have seen a remarkable increase in our members training proficiency. It was definitely the right decision to have you come and train my members. Once again my heartfelt appreciation for sharing your knowledge and expertise with us and increasing our likelihood of surviving a situation with the enemy in our future missions.

> —**John J. Chianese**, Lt. Col. NYANG, Commander Security Forces, Department of the Air Force.

Your training and skills greatly assisted our Marines by allowing them to successfully learn a valuable combat skill set that will continue to serve the Marines for the remainder of their careers and enhance their warrior ethos. It is with the utmost pleasure that I express to you my personal gratitude and appreciation for a job well done.

> —**M.K. Jeron**, Major, United States Marine Corps.

Your krav maga instruction significantly enhanced the soldiers' knowledge of hand to hand combat, weapons defense, straight edge and firearms combat, and defense fighting techniques. Your efforts and dedication reflects distinct credit upon yourself and the Israeli Krav Maga Association.

—**Peter R. Mucciarone**, Lt. Col., Department of the Army.

On the behalf of the men and women of the Joint Base Police Department, 87th Security Forces Squadron. … I would like to extend a sincere thanks for the time, combat-proven skills and dedication that you have unselfishly bestowed on the following courses: (1) Terror and Active Shooter Attack Intervention; (2) Aircraft Assault and Takeover; (3) IKMA Israeli Krav Maga Instructor Course; (4) RAVEN Krav Maga. I have met with dozens of Tactical/Combatives Trainers trying to produce this, but you were the only team with an IDF Special Operations background … This was money well spent because I cannot put a price on the lives of my Airmen, Sailors and Police Officers! A stellar referral from the NJSP Director himself put you over the top! Thank you!

—**David A. Haigh**, Major, USAF, Operations Officer, Department of the Air Force, Joint Base McGuire-Dix-Lakehurst.

David Kahn and his associate instructors were professionals who took the mission accomplishment and instruction to a whole new level. I have been doing martial arts over 22 years and honestly say that Krav Maga is the single most effective fighting system … Krav Maga allows both armed and unarmed combat to flow from the same basic instinctual movements making it perfect for the military, law enforcement professional, or the professional housewife. Krav Maga is a simple system with brutal effectiveness. I would recommend David Kahn and this program to any organization looking for a time and cost effective program.

—**T.J. Ardese**, Lt. Col., United States Marine Corps.

KRAV MAGA

WEAPON DEFENSES

KRAV MAGA

WEAPON DEFENSES

DAVID KAHN

THE CONTACT COMBAT SYSTEM OF THE ISRAEL DEFENSE FORCES

YMAA Publication Center
Wolfeboro, N.H., USA

YMAA Publication Center, Inc.
PO Box 480
Wolfeboro, NH 03894
800 669-8892 • www.ymaa.com • info@ymaa.com

Paperback
ISBN: 978-1-59439-240-5

Ebook
ISBN: 978-1-59439-242-9

Cover design by Axie Breen
Editing by Susan Bullowa
Front cover photo by Rinaldo Rossi

10 9 8 7 6 5 4 3 2

Publisher's Cataloging in Publication

Kahn, David, 1972-

Krav maga weapon defenses / by David Kahn. – Wolfeboro, NH :
YMAA Publication Center, c2012.

p. ; cm.

ISBN: 978-1-59439-240-5 (pbk.) ; 978-1-59439-242-9 (ebk.)
Includes bibliographical references and index.
Contents: Introduction – Control holds reviewed – Impact weapon defenses – Leg defenses against edged-weapon attacks – Hand defenses against edged weapons – Handgun defenses – Rifle/submachine gun (SMG) defenses – Kravist weapon defense drills – Appendix: vehicle safety tips, road rage, and carjacking – Index – Biographies – Resources.

1. Krav maga. 2. Self-defense. 3. Hand-to-hand fighting. 4. Martial arts–Training. I. Title.

GV1111 .K248 2012   2012938841
796.81–dc23   1206

Warning: While self-defense is legal, fighting is illegal. If you don't know the difference you'll go to jail because you aren't defending yourself, you are fighting—or worse. Readers are encouraged to be aware of all appropriate local and national laws relating to self-defense, reasonable force, and the use of weaponry, and act in accordance with all applicable laws at all times. Understand that while legal definitions and interpretations are generally uniform, there are small—but very important—differences from state to state. To stay out of jail, you need to know these differences. Neither the author nor the publisher assumes any responsibility for the use or misuse of information contained in this book.

Nothing in this document constitutes a legal opinion nor should any of its contents be treated as such. While the author believes that everything herein is accurate, any questions regarding specific self-defense situations, legal liability, and/or interpretation of federal, state, or local laws should always be addressed by an attorney at law. This text relies on public news sources to gather information on various crimes and criminals described herein. While news reports of such incidences are generally accurate, they are on occasion incomplete or incorrect. Consequently, all suspects should be considered innocent until proven guilty in a court of law.

When it comes to martial arts, self-defense, and related topics, no text, no matter how well written, can substitute for professional, hands-on instruction. These materials should be used **for academic study only**.

Table of Contents

Dedication

For Claire, Benjamin, and Leo
In Loving Memory of Helen Brener Smith

Acknowledgements

I am indebted to Grandmaster **Haim Gidon** for instilling Israeli krav maga at its highest and most evolved level. As head of the Israeli krav maga system and President of the Israeli Krav Maga Association (IKMA Gidon System), Haim continues to develop and improve krav maga with the blessing of **Imi Litchtenfeld**, its founder. I am grateful to my other Israeli krav maga instructors and close friends, the **Gidon** family, **Yoav Krayn** and family, **Yigal Arbiv, Eran Buaron, Itzik Cohen**, and **Steve Moishe. Aldema Tzrinksky** is a great friend providing immeasurable support and counsel over the many years. I am grateful to the **Hauerstocks** for their sabra hospitality in my bi-annual visits to Israel and my good friend **Shira Orbas** now one of the best in the security "business" along with her wonderful family. I offer special thanks to Master **Kobi Lichtenstein** and his organization for their hospitality.

Sgt. Major (Res.) **Nir Maman**, former lead counter terror and krav maga instructor for the Israel Defense Force's Counter Terror School (LOTAR) and IDF Infantry and Paratroopers Ground Forces Command Soldier of the Year 2009, has provided great support, professional insights, and specialized training expertise as only he can. Former krav maga chief military instructor **Boaz Aviram** and former lead combat instructor **Shay Amir** are great and appreciated resources. Major **David Hasid**, the IKMA Board of Directors and all IKMA members who continue to welcome and train with me over the years. Yet again, this book would not be possible without the expert training, support, and inspiration of krav maga's backbone: the IKMA (www.kravmagaisraeli.com).

This book would not exist without senior krav maga instructors **Rick Blitstein** and **Alan Feldman.** Rick and Alan are redoubts of support and reservoirs of knowledge. Their wisdom makes me a better instructor and person. I am indebted to all my friend krav maga friends, supporters, network, and fellow instructors **Rinaldo Rossi, Mike Delahanty, David Ordini, Avital Zeisler, Jeff Gorman, Don Melnick, David Gollin, Pat Smullen, George Foster, Jose Anaya, Thom Farrel, Jason Bleitstein, Bert Witte, Frank Colluci, Mike Bottone, Jesse Dunn, Joe Tucker, Rich Felsher, Chris Dawson, David Rahn, John Hartmann, Chris Morrison, Elizabeth Greenman, Robb Hamic, Al Ackerman, Greg Holland, Tray Hallman**, along with all those instructors about to join us. I give special thanks to **Chris Eckel** for his great help and unparalleled support. Our friends in Poland and Portugal, **Kris Sawicki** and **Vitor Martin,** keep the IKMA at the forefront in Europe. I am grateful to all our students both in New York City and at our New Jersey based Israeli Krav Maga United States Training Centers (www.israelikrav.com).

Thanks to **A.B. Duki** and **Marc** of the Residence Beach Hotel (www.zyvotels.com) for hosting our bi-annual training stays in Netanya. **A.J. Yolofsky** and **Enrique Prado** deserve thanks for their public support and efforts. I am also grateful to **Kim** and **Oliver Pimley** for their dedication and **Art Co** for his support and explaining the nuances of Philippine edged-weapons tactics. The **Tenenbaums** and **Goldbergs** remain pillars of my life and mishpacha. I am grateful to **Bill Kingson** for his continued support. I would like to give special thanks to **James Gandolfini**, **Richard Miller**, and **John Mayer** for their trust and backing.

A special thanks on both a personal and professional level to all of our friends and supporters in the law enforcement community including **Lt. Miller**, **Sgt. McComb**, **Sgt. Klem**, **Sgt. Oehlman**, **Lt. Maimone**, **Lt. Ponetti**, **Capt. Savalli** (Ret.), **Associate Director Harrison**, **Chief Lazzarotti**, **Director Paglione**, **Investigators Smith and Gioscio**, **Officer Fleher**, **Officer Tucker**, **Officer Hanafee**, **Lt. Colon**, **Sgt. Hayden**, **Officer Davis**, **Officer Johnson**, **Special Agent-in-Charge Hammond** and **Special Agents Schroeder** and **Belle**, **Special Agents Clark**, **Di Cola** and **Nowazcek**, **Special Agents Smith**, **Canestrari**, and **Crowe**, along with the many other law enforcement professionals with whom we have the honor of working, especially, **Officer Fetzer**.

Lastly, I would like to thank the following United States Marine Corps personnel: **Capt. Small** (Ret.), **Maj. "Sparky" Bollinger**, **GySgt. Jacobs**, **Sgts. Ladler**, **Parker**, and **Allen**, **Lt. Col. "Tonto" Ardese**, **SSgt. Jensen**, **Cpl. Lackland**, **SSgt. Kropelwicki**, **MGySgt. (Ret.) Urso** along with **Maj. Haigh** of the United States Air Force, and **1Sg. Johnson**, for their support along to all of our fighting men and women of the United States military and Israel Defense Forces for safeguarding our freedom. Security expert **Steven Hartov**, one of my favorite authors and good friends, deserves much gratitude for his personal and professional support. I am grateful to Drs. **Steven Gecha**, **Stephen Hunt**, and **Bruce Rose**, and PTs **Lindsey Balint** and **Jeff Manheimer** continue to hold me together. Thanks to **Jerry Palmieri** for his conditioning advice along with **George Samuelson** and **"Doc" Mark Cheng**.

My family serves as a buttress and the wellspring of support, especially my wife Claire, for the growth of krav maga training and for being the bastion of support for our expansion. I am grateful to my uncle Harry and stepfather Ed for their unwavering support. My father, Alfred, and mother, Anne, always saw the brutal logic. My brother, Abel, is uniquely capable. Benjamin and Leo are our future.

I offer special thanks to my good friend and one-of-a-kind photographer **Ed Greenblatt**. This book would not exist without his dedication, patience, and generosity, along with that of my instructors and business partners **Rinaldo Rossi**, **Don Melnick**, **Avital Zeisler**, **James Gandolfi**, **John Mayer**, and **Richard Miller**.

I am especially grateful to my Publisher **David Ripianzi** for recognizing the need for a book featuring the latest evolution of Israeli krav maga weapon defenses along with his professional insights and allowing us to present nearly 800 photos. My editor, **Susan Bullowa**, deserves a heartfelt thank you for her herculean effort and dedication to policing this manuscript and whipping it into top form. *Kol ha kavod*, Susan!

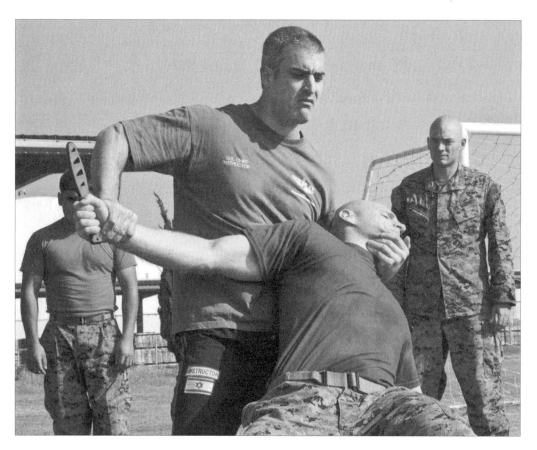

Training U.S. Marines. Photo courtesy of USMC Combat Camera.

Introduction

Before we explore specific defenses in the chapters, there are several principles to keep in mind.

The Language of Krav Maga

Throughout *Krav Maga Weapon Defenses*, the following terms will appear frequently. Once you understand the language of *krav maga* (means *contact combat* in Hebrew), you can then better understand the method.

"Negative Five." You are caught unaware and at a complete disadvantage. The attacker has the advantage of surprise and positioning.

Combative. Any manner of strike, takedown, throw, joint lock, choke, or other offensive fighting movement.

Retzev. A Hebrew word that means "continuous motion" in combat. Retzev, the backbone of modern Israeli krav maga, teaches you to move your body instinctively in combat motion without thinking about your next move. When in a dangerous situation, you will automatically call upon your physical and mental training to a launch seamless overwhelming counterattack, using strikes, takedowns, throws, joint locks, chokes or other offensive actions combined with evasive action. Retzev is quick and decisive movement merging all aspects of your krav maga training. Defensive movements transition automatically into offensive movements to neutralize the attack, affording your opponent little time to react.

Left outlet stance. Blades your body by turning your feet approximately 30 degrees to your right, with your left arm and left leg forward. (You can also turn 30 degrees to your right to come into a right regular outlet stance, so that your right leg and arm are forward.) You are resting on the ball of your rear foot in a comfortable and balanced position. Your feet should be parallel with about 55 percent of your weight distributed over your front leg. Your arms are positioned in front of your face and bent slightly forward at approximately a 60-degree angle between your forearms and your upper arms. From this stance, move forward, laterally, and backward, moving your feet in concert.

Liveside. When you are facing the front of your opponent and your opponent can both see you and use all four arms and legs against you, you are facing his or her liveside.

Deadside. Your opponent's deadside, in contrast to his liveside, places you behind his near shoulder or facing his back. You are in an advantageous position to counterattack and control him because it is difficult for him to use his arm and leg farthest away from you to attack you. You should always move to the deadside when possible. This also places the opponent between you and any additional third-party threat.

Sameside. Your sameside arm or leg faces your opponent when you are positioned opposite one another. For example, if you are directly facing your opponent and your right side is opposite your opponent's left side, your sameside arm is your right arm (opposite his left arm).

Nearside. Your opponent's limb closest to your torso.

Outside defense. An outside defense counters an outside attack, that is, an attack directed at you from the outside of your body to the inside. A slap to the face or hook punch are examples of outside attacks.

Inside defense. An inside defense defends against an inside or straight attack. This type of attack involves a thrusting motion, such as jabbing your finger into someone's eye or punching someone in the nose.

Glicha. A Hebrew term meaning a sliding movement on the balls of your feet to carry your entire bodyweight forward and through a combative strike to maximize its impact.

Secoul. A Hebrew term meaning a larger step than glicha, covering more distance to carry your entire bodyweight forward and through a combative strike to maximize its impact.

Off-angle. An attack angle that is not face-to-face.

Stepping off the line. Use footwork and body movement to take evasive action against a linear attack, such as a straight punch or kick. Such movement is also referred to as "breaking the angle of attack."

Tsai-bake. A Japanese term meaning a one-hundred-eighty-degree or semi-circle step by rotating one leg back to create torque on a joint to complete a takedown or control hold.

Cavalier. A wrist takedown forcing an adversary's wrist to move against its natural range of motion usually combined with tsai-bake for added power.

Elbow kiss. When securing an edged weapon or firearm held by an assailant and pinning it against the his body, the defender moves to the assailant's deadside creating an angle between the defender's arm and assailant's arm where the tips of their respective elbows touch or "kiss." The defender's forearm and assailant's gun arm create a "V" by the underside of your forearm pressing against the topside of the assailant's forearm

Trapping. Occurs when you pin or grab the opponent's arms with one arm, leaving you with free to continue combatives with your other arm.

Figure Four. A control hold securing an opponent's arm, torso, or ankle to exert pressure. The control hold is enabled by using both of your arms on the joint of the wrist, shoulder, or tendon of an opponent. For example, you have secured your opponent's right wrist (his elbow is pointed toward the ground) with your right hand placed on the flat of his right hand, bending his wrist inward, with his elbow (tip toward the ground) pinned to your chest while you simultaneously slip your other arm over the top of his forearm to interlock his arm and grab your own forearm. This positional arm control may also be used to attack the Achilles tendon with the blade of your forearm or control an opponent's torso from the rearmount. A Figure Four may also be applied to an opponent's torso by hooking one leg across the torso and securing it in the crook of the other leg's knee.

Kravist. A term I coined to describe a smart and prepared krav maga fighter.

Cold Weapons. Blunt and edged weapons.

Hot Weapons. Firearms.

Kimura. Armlock named after its inventor, Masahiko Kimura.

Street Violence

Street violence is, by its nature, volatile and unpredictable. To be sure, there are no certainties, especially regarding the outcome of a life and death struggle. The last thing on many victims' minds is that they will be battered, clubbed, stabbed, slashed, or shot. Oftentimes, you will find yourself in a "negative five" position or initially unprepared to fight for your life. An attacker will seek every advantage. First and foremost, he will try to use the element of surprise, especially, to deploy a weapon.

In 2010, the Federal Bureau of Investigation estimated 1,246,248 violent crimes nationwide.

- Aggravated assaults (defined by the FBI as "as an unlawful attack by one person upon another for the purpose of inflicting severe or aggravated bodily injury") accounted for the highest number of violent crimes reported to law enforcement at 62.5 percent. Of this 62.5 percent of aggravated assaults, firearms were used 20.6 percent; knives/cutting instruments 19.0 percent; clubs/blunt objects 33.1 percent; and personal weapons for 27.4 percent of reported cases.

- Robbery comprised 29.5 percent of violent crimes. Of this 29.5 percent, firearms were used 41.4 percent; while strong-arm tactics were used 42.0 percent; followed by knives and cutting instruments 7.9 percent; and other dangerous weapons 8.8 percent of the reported cases.

- Murder accounted for 1.2 percent of estimated violent crimes in 2010. Of this 1.2 percent; firearms were used 67.5 percent; knives/cutting instruments 13.1 percent; other weapons 13.6 percent; and personal weapons for 6.6 percent of reported cases.

- Forcible rape accounted for 6.8 percent of reported violent crime. Reported statistics do not account for the criminal use of weapons, but, past FBI surveys have indicated that approximately 10–20 percent of forcible annual rapes involve the use of a weapon.

- Source: Federal Bureau of Investigation Uniform Crime Reporting (UCR) Program 2010. For the most current information visit www.fbi.gov.

- In a 2010 National Crime Victimization Survey compiled by the Bureau of Justice Statistics, 852,660 specific weapon related violent crimes were reported in the United States. Of these 852,660 violent victimizations:
- 337,960 violent crimes were committed with firearms
- 192,320 violent crimes were committed with knives
- 266,620 violent crimes were committed with "other" and "unknown" weapons

In this study, the ratio of simple and aggravated weapon related assaults (616,670 incidents) compared to armed robberies (212,390 incidents) was roughly 3:1. Accordingly, one can extrapolate that when a weapon was present, a victim was three times more likely to be physically attacked rather then simply threatened.

Source: For the most current information visit www. bjs.ojp.usdoj.gov.

Criminals who use weapons are often not particularly well trained. For example, a controlled pull on the trigger of a firearm versus a hard pull is not something the average criminal gunman spends much time contemplating let alone practicing. Staving your skull versus simply knocking you unconscious is also a *non-acquired skill*. He may not know the fine line between knocking you unconscious and killing you. An armed assailant's judgment may also be impaired by an admixture of inebriation, mental illness, or any other human emotion giving vent to violent rage.

Violence is an ugly grisly affair. If you are threatened or attacked, the assailant thinks he can win. You cannot doubt the assailant is committed, through violence, to dominating or destroying you. He is willing to cause you egregious, perhaps deadly, bodily harm by eviscerating, puncturing or spilling your internal organs, shattering bones, or pulping your brain. When unexpectedly caught in the sites of a deranged attacker or psychopathic predator, you may wonder, "Why is this stranger attacking me?" This thinking may occur continue, for example, even after the third, fourth, or fifth stab wounds of the ambush. This is why you must hone your mental to physical skills until you can call on them without thinking. With enough practice, you will train to react instinctively and swiftly. Only proper training can trigger this fighting response. Realistic training improves this reaction flow by allowing you to quickly assess violent situations and react under stress.

Training ingrains the appropriate responses into your memory bank improving your reaction time. Whether the threat comes from an edged weapon or gun, you will already know how to react. Equally important, proper training compels the most suitable reaction for a given situation. An attack launched by surprise will force you to react from an unprepared state. Therefore, your self-defense reaction must be instinctive and reflexive. Krav maga training prepares you for just that. Your subconscious mind will turn your instinctive trained responses into immediate action. Instinct assumes control. This autonomic response is vital because your instantaneous reaction will occur just prior to your natural adrenaline dump that can momentarily or permanently interfere with your fine and gross motor skills—your defensive capability. In other words, optimally, you won't have time to think. You'll make the defense before you even realize what is happening just as your adrenaline dump reaches its apex.

One of the most effective tactics krav maga can teach you is not to be taken by surprise in the first place. Developing recognition of pre-violence indicators along with impending attack identification skills are instrumental to krav maga training. Once you develop an awareness of your environment—any environment—you will notice at all times who and what surrounds you. By recognizing a potential threat, such as the bulge of a handgun sequestered in a waistband, before the assailant can deploy it, you can avoid a life-threatening situation. The best defense against any attack is removing yourself from the situation before the attack can take place. Only awareness of your environment can help you do that.

Situational awareness is all-important and common sense should prevail. In an unknown environment, keep your head subtly swiveling by shifting your eye movements, using your peripheral vision, and panning for potential threats. Constantly survey your surroundings. In a worrisome situation, always watch a suspicious person's hand movement. Let's say you are watching a potential adversary's hand movements. You notice that the hands are hidden in a pocket about to pull out a weapon—stop him. Along the same lines, recognition of a bulge on a potential assailant's body—a possible weapon—also allows you to take the initiative.

Remember, a weapon can be sequestered in many places and concealed from view even when an assailant is grasping it. Krav maga trainees scrutinize how someone can conceal a weapon, such as holding an edged weapon in a reverse grip with the blade parallel to the forearm and shielded from view. An impact weapon, edged weapon, or firearm could be placed behind an assailant's leg ready for immediate use. Also sensitize your hearing for clues such as the lock-back of a folding edged-weapon clicking or the sound of a round being chambered in a firearm. Awareness and mental conditioning are integral to krav maga training.

Other indicators might be someone who seems distinctly out of place, loitering, or who is mirroring or following your movements. Criminals can telegraph their intent through nervous or abnormal behavior leading up to an attack. It cannot be emphasized enough the need to watch a suspicious person's hands. A hand concealing a weapon will usually be stiff, contorted, or move in an unnatural way. This can be particularly noticeable when a potentially dangerous person is approaching you and his arms swing or don't swing—another indicator. If someone's arms are crossed concealing the hands, you should also take note. In addition, an assailant could also distract you by speaking to you, or asking you question such as the time to force you to look at your watch, phone, etc. to catch you by surprise while he simultaneously presents a weapon to threaten or attack you. Be especially aware of someone turning his back to you in close proximity as he pulls his hands in front of his torso; another preferred stealth method for weapon deployment.

Three seminal works, *Meditations on Violence* (YMAA 2008) and *Facing Violence* (YMAA 2011) both by Rory Miller along with *The Little Black Book of Violence* by Lawrence Kane and Kris Wilder (YMAA 2009), provide comprehensive insights into the psychology and physiology of violence. Reading these works will further develop an understanding of street violence's underpinnings. Each of these works also provides a strong foundation for how to best extricate yourself from harm's way before you have no choice but to engage in counter-violence. Many of these authors' key points dovetail extremely well with the krav maga's holistic self-defense approach:

• Understanding the warning signs of impending violence
• How predators operate
• The brutal reality of a violent encounter
• Violence's aftermath including first aid and legal redress or ramifications

To harm you with an edged or impact weapon, an attacker must close the distance. To have better accuracy with a firearm, an attacker may also close the distance. If you see the attacker brandishing a weapon before he can close on you, naturally you would try to escape when possible. The assailant usually knows this and will conceal the weapon until the opportune moment to present it. In addition, a criminally-minded assailant would prefer not to have witnesses or as few as possible up until the very last moment of the attack. Note: If you witness a crime, you may be the next victim because the attacker wishes to eliminate anyone who can identify him.

Human Emotional Responses in a Life-threatening Encounter

One of my best friends, Sgt. Major Nir Maman (res.), provides a superb explanation of the range of human emotional responses when encountering a life-threatening encounter:

"Do not become a victim of shock. When confronting a life-threatening situation, shock can be more of a problem than fear. If you go into shock while under attack, you will freeze and not do anything. The reason people go into shock when attacked is a lack of response preparation. The mind is divided into two sections, the conscious mind, and the subconscious mind.

"The conscious mind is your cognitive thinking process. The conscious mind engages when you have the time to assess a situation thoroughly and respond deliberately. If you are caught off guard and are overwhelmed with

stress, your conscious mind shuts down and transfers all thought process to your subconscious mind.

"This happens because your mind does not have the time to thoroughly go through its four steps of reaction due to the overload of information and stress. The mind short circuits and shuts down. Your subconscious mind is nothing more than an instinctive response command or a data bank of muscle memory. If your subconscious mind has no concrete muscle memory stored to engage the immediate problem, it simply makes your body defend itself the best way it knows how. Often, this is to throw your arms up in front of your face and chest to protect the body's vital areas and crouch down to become a smaller target.

"If your subconscious muscle memory cannot summon an instinctive response, your conscious mind will still make your body respond with its own primitive defenses described above. Instincts will always dominate over cognitive response under stress.

"You may be familiar with the expression 'I saw my life flash in front of my eyes.' Many people experience this response when they are in a situation where they think they are about to die. This response happens for a very specific reason that is geared at helping you survive under stress. The reason you see your life flash in front of your eyes is simple. When overwhelming stress shuts down your cognitive or conscious mind, responsibility transfers over to your subconscious mind. If your subconscious mind has no proper muscle memory stored, it is confounded with no solution. Your subconscious mind scans the entire data bank of your life, from the day you were born to the present second, to evaluate if you were ever in a similar situation and how you responded. If there was a similar or parallel situation, your subconscious mind will take that same response and implement it to the current situation to help you survive.

"To avoid going into shock under stress, like in the training to deal with fear, constantly visualize yourself in every possible attack situation you may find yourself in and train yourself over and over in your mind until you have effective solutions for those situations."

Sgt. Major Nir Maman (res.) served in the Israeli Special Forces (ISF) Central Command Counter Terror and Hostage Rescue Unit and the Special Forces Counter Terror and Special Operations School (CTSO) Nir's duties included training the CTSO's instructors in CT Warfare, Tactical Shooting, and krav maga. He also held the Lead Counter Terror Instructor position on the CTSO's designated Hostage Rescue Take-Over

(HRT) Units Instructor Team, where he was responsible for training new recruits and active operational members of the ISF's designated HRT units in all areas of counter terror warfare and hostage rescue including hostage rescue operations in friendly and hostile/foreign environments; close-quarters combat; dynamic entry; aircraft, ship, train, and bus interdiction; suicide bomber interception; urban warfare; tactical shooting; and krav maga. In April 2009, Nir was awarded the IDF Ground Forces Infantry and Ground Forces Command Soldier of the Year Award of Excellence.

In the case of an edged-weapon attack, there is a good chance if someone attacks you by surprise, you will see an arm movement, but you may not always see the weapon. To be sure, running away from a threat or impending attack is a real and sensible option. Do not let ego, a sense of indignity, or just plain anger get you seriously hurt or killed. Of course, there are circumstances when you cannot run, such as being with family or friends who are not mobile. You will have to stand your ground and defend.

Realistic physical training, along with mental training to envision different kinds of attacks, regulates your response. Training "hardwires" your brain to move your body instinctively to bypass conscious thought and streamline the self-defense process: to think without thinking. The self-defense process may be understood by using the following four-part process:

1) Threat recognition
2) Situation analysis
3) Choice of action
4) Action or inaction

Krav maga's goal is to embed your subconscious with the proverbial "[I have] been there done that (through a training scenario)." Most important, you should have confidence in your krav maga training because all techniques are battle-tested and field-proven. Do not, however, mistake your training for a real attack. In an actual attack, you will experience an adrenaline surge, a likely decrease in your fine motor skills, your heart rate will skyrocket, your hearing will diminish ("auditory exclusion"), and your vision will narrow (often known as "tunnel vision").

Notably, most people who have survived violent confrontations had the mental commitment to prevail. They do not often attribute their survival to a specific technique. With this in mind, krav maga provides latitude in its techniques, and flexibility in its thinking. In a successful defense, while there may an optimum tactic and strategy, if the defender survives, optimally unscathed, his krav maga worked. Critically important in defending weapons: You do not have the latitude for error that defending an unarmed attack might allow. Technique deficiency can get you seriously injured or killed.

Krav Maga's Methodology

The essence of Israeli krav maga is to neutralize an opponent quickly. There are no rules in an unscripted fight, especially in an armed confrontation. This lack of rules distinguishes self-defense from sport fighting. To stop an assailant, krav maga primarily targets the body's vital soft tissue, chiefly the groin, neck, and eyes. Other secondary targets include the kidneys, solar plexus, knees, liver, joints, fingers, nerve centers, and other smaller fragile bones. In addition, krav maga teaches you to disarm the assailant and, if necessary, turn the weapon against your assailant. Krav maga differs from other self-defense systems that may rely primarily on targeting difficult to locate nerve centers. In the heat of a violent struggle, this type of precise counterattack strategy is extremely difficult. Conversely, a krav maga combative to the groin or strong combative to the head is precise enough to debilitate the opponent while simple to deliver.

When defending against weapons and escape is not possible, krav maga's essential philosophy is to close the distance between the defender and assailant to neutralize the weapon and, whenever possible, take the defender out of the "line of fire."

Optimally, the distance between the defender and the assailant can be closed before a weapon is deployed while simultaneously debilitating the adversary with strong combatives, blocking access to the weapon, and achieving dominant control. If the weapon is successfully deployed and put into action, closing the distance allows the defender to deflect-redirect or block the weapon, the majority of time in combination with body defenses while delivering withering counterattacks.

The Israeli krav maga fighting system is designed to work against any attacker. The key is your mindset. As my good friend Nir Maman, Lead Counter Terror Instructor for the Israel Defense Force, explains so well, you must be able to transition from a highly disadvantageous "negative five" position to an advantageous "positive five" position instinctively and instantaneously. You must turn the table on your opponent(s) immediately. Self-preservation is a powerful motivator—so is protecting others. If you must defend yourself, you need to dominate your attacker and incapacitate him. Krav maga's core techniques provide cumulative building blocks for a formidable self-defense foundation. A few mastered techniques go a long way and are highly effective against weapon threats and attacks.

Krav maga's defensive philosophy is never to do more than necessary, but to react instinctively with speed, economy of motion, and the appropriate measure of force. Instinctive reaction is paramount and you are taught to strike instinctively at the human body's vulnerable parts. Israeli krav maga training tries to place you in the most realistic training scenarios including weapon attacks with all possible attendant variations. The goal is to present instinctive solutions to overcome threats and defeat deadly attacks. Krav maga uses the same building blocks from the simplest defenses to the most advanced techniques, including empty-handed defenses, and disarms against bladed weapons, firearms, and even micro-explosives, as you will soon learn. Most important, krav maga emphasizes that there are no rules on the street. If a situation is dire, do whatever is necessary to overcome the threat.

A trainee immediately appreciates krav maga's simplicity and universal applicability. Krav maga uses the concept of retzev, Hebrew for "continuous motion" to complete a defense. Retzev, the backbone of modern Israeli krav maga, teaches you to move your body instinctively in combat motion without thinking about your next move. Training becomes first nature rather than second nature. When in a dangerous situation, you will automatically call upon your physical and mental training to a launch seamless overwhelming counterattack using strikes, takedowns, throws, joint locks, chokes, or other offensive actions combined with evasive action. Retzev is quick and decisive movement merging all aspects of your krav maga training. Defensive movements transition automatically into offensive movements to neutralize the attack affording your opponent little time to react.

Imi summarized, "it [defensive movements] comes from the head." Your brain absorbs, retains, translates, and harnesses your instincts to launch your body into action. Keep in mind that two attacks will be delivered in the same manner. Defenders are given tools for their toolboxes along with a general blueprint how to use them. Remember, Imi's goal was survival in any defensible situation. You must develop a strong understanding and grasp of how and why you might find yourself embroiled in a violent encounter. How did he (the assailant) get so close to me without my noticing? Was he acting aggressively toward others before he turned on me? Am I a specific target or a random target put in harm's way by bad luck?

To make the method yours and react instinctively, you must put just as much emphasis on mental training as you do the physical. In a potential deadly force confrontation, you may experience a combined surge of stress, fear, and excitement. When you are fearful, the nervous system increases the body's physical capabilities by injecting adrenaline into the blood stream. Although fear helps you to survive by quickening your heart rate and sending more oxygenated blood to your muscles, you must harness your fear and remain levelheaded. You must control involuntary body responses, such as quivering legs, to execute the correct self-defense reactions. You will need both physical and mental training to learn how to harness this fear-induced adrenaline surge.

Mental and physical conditioning allows you to harness your adrenaline and channel it into action. Mental confidence and toughness, in particular, provides a decisive advantage in a violent encounter. When you feel confident, you believe that your training will carry the day regardless of an opponent's possession of a weapon. Confidence, however, must not lead to overconfidence. Do not underestimate the opponent, especially, when he has the mechanical advantage of a weapon. And, always expect the unexpected.

Mental conditioning will help build your confidence, preventing the panic that can lead to freezing or poor decision making. Mental conditioning will also allow you to de-escalate or walk away (always the best solution if possible) from a potentially a violent situation.

With proper training, you will learn how to use fear and other negative emotions to your advantage. You will harness the energy and power from your body's fight or flight response rather than freezing under pressure. If you merely read through this book but do not actually train against impact weapons, edged weapons, and firearm threats on a regular basis, physical trauma coupled with fright and shock will most likely negate rational thought, paralyzing you into inaction. When in danger, the brain searches its memory bank for a response. In a violent encounter, if an opponent takes an unanticipated or unrecognized action, the brain cannot find a practiced response resulting in decision paralysis. Denial is the most common obstacle to taking appropriate action. Often, with an untrained mind and body, it is difficult to process or accept that someone else intends you serious bodily harm. An assailant may know this and achieve his purpose accordingly.

Krav maga's goal is to make a trainee proficient in defending himself or herself against any manner of attack in the shortest possible training period. As krav maga is based on our most primitive and natural instincts, a few core defensive movements harnessing gross motor skills can be learned, retained, and applied to overcome numerous deadly force threats while under duress. For example, the same defensive movement can defend against a hook punch, an overhand, forward slash, or a hook stab to the throat or head. This training principle is crucial: good defensive tactics training should rely on a few instinctive and adaptable core techniques.

In krav maga, you will learn a few elementary techniques that you can perform instinctively and apply to a wide variety of situations. You will learn how to protect your vital points and organs. Equally important, you will know how to debilitate an opponent by striking his or her vital anatomy. If the situation requires, krav maga will teach you how to maximize the damage you can inflict by striking, kneeing, kicking, chopping, gouging, choking, dislocating joints, breaking bones, and taking your opponent down to the ground.

You need not master hundreds of self-defense techniques to become a kravist or competent krav maga fighter capable of defeating an armed attack or threat. Non-violent conflict resolution is always your best solution. In krav maga, we prepare for any type and number of attacks and threats. While there are no set solutions for ending an armed confrontation, there are preferred methods using retzev or "continuous combat motion" to prevail. When defending against weapons, retzev is modified ("modified weapons retzev") because the nearside arm often controls the attacker's weapon or weapon arm. Combined with simultaneous defense and attack, retzev is a seamless, decisive, and overwhelming counterattack forming the backbone of the Israeli fighting system.

Retzev can be understood using combined upper- and lower-body combatives, locks, chokes, throws, takedowns, and weapons interchangeably without pause.

The human body can withstand a high degree of physical punishment. Certain attacks can be lethal, but even when severely injured, the body can perform nearly miraculous feats. Adrenaline is a powerful energizer and allows the body to momentarily insulate itself against pain. The body's resilience works for both victim and assailant. Note that an assailant under the influence of drugs acquires yet another layer of pain insulation and artificially increased strength.

Keep in mind, however, that the level of force you use to defend yourself should be commensurate with the threat. Developed as a military fighting discipline, krav maga employs lethal force techniques. When faced with a deadly force encounter, you may, in turn, need to employ lethal counterforce. Forging an awareness of your own personal weapons (hands, forearms, elbows, knees, shins, feet, and head) and an opponent's vulnerabilities is essential to fight strategy and tactics, especially when he is armed and you are not. As noted, the human body is amazingly resilient, even when subjected to tremendous physical abuse. Pain may stop some attackers, but other individuals have enormous pain thresholds, especially those taking narcotics.

Krav Maga Tactics

Once engaged against an assailant, the key to all krav maga weapons defenses is a deflection-redirection of the weapon combined with a simultaneous body defense and an overwhelming counterattack. This methodology is designed to stop the attack at its inception, or at the earliest possible stage. Closing the distance gap between the assailant and defender is sometimes referred to as "bursting." The opposite of bursting forward is a bursting retreat to escape or create distance until the correct time to close the gap presents itself. Counterattacks usually target the assailant's soft tissue including his groin, throat, eyes, and knees. Weapon defenses take into specific account the assailant's physiological reaction to counterstrikes such as a knee or kick to the groin that will lurch the body forward or a thumb gouge to the eye that will jolt the head back exposing the groin for further strikes.

Footwork and body positioning, whether standing or prone, allow you to simultaneously defend and attack, leading to seamless combative transitions essential to retzev. Good balance is a must with your weight properly positioned on the balls of your feet to react; not on your heels. Balance within any stance is essential to redirect your energy and momentum. A good stance, either from the left outlet position or even from a passive stance, allows you to press directly into the ground for superior traction and mobility. Accordingly, if you have good balance and mobility, you can burst in to close on the assailant. The key to evasion is moving out of the "line of fire" or the path of an opponent's offensive combatives. Clearly, positioning yourself where you can counterattack your opponent more easily than he can attack you is most advantageous.

Essential to a successful defense is precise fight timing: using the correct tactic at the correct time. Fight timing is best thought of as the fusion of instinct with simultaneous decision-making to either preempt the attack, move off the line of attack/fire, deflect-redirect, control the weapon and strike, or to retreat from harm's way. In other words, fight timing is harnessing instinctive body movements while seizing or creating opportunities to defend both efficiently and intelligently.

Defined yet another way, fight timing is your ability to capitalize on a window of opportunity offered by your opponent or to create your own opportunity to end the confrontation, using whatever tactics come instinctively to you. Timing can be improved and honed with realistic training—always krav maga's objective. While speed is not timing, speed certainly can add a decisive advantage when the defender is faster than the assailant. As the subsequent chapters emphasize, krav maga relies on economy of motion to eliminate wasted movement, which, in turn, improves speed.

Footwork and body positioning, whether standing or prone, allow you to simultaneously defend and attack, providing for the seamless combative transitions essential to retzev. The key to evasion is moving out of the "line of fire" or the path of an assailant's weapon. Clearly, controlling the weapon and positioning yourself where you can counterattack your opponent more easily than he can attack you is optimum.

A punch thrown at your head does not represent the same danger, as does an edged weapon slashing at your throat. Countering an open-handed strike to your head by deflecting-redirecting the attack and simultaneously collapsing your attacker's windpipe may not be justified under these circumstances (although, of course, the totality of the circumstances must always be taken into consideration). However, when someone tries to slit your throat, you are justified in stopping the deadly force assault as quickly as possible using any means at your disposal. This particular defense against an edged-weapon attack to the head involves the defender stepping "off the line" of attack and simultaneously counterstriking the assailant in the face or throat as we will cover in Chapter 4.

Defending against this same example of a face-to-face overhand edged-weapon attack (often called an icepick attack) also serves as a good example how krav maga incorporates open-handed defensive tactics with tactical positioning to put

Krav Maga Tactical Thinking When Confronting Weapons While on the Ground. One of the best ways to stop a weapon from being deployed in a ground struggle is exactly that: prevent the assailant from presenting the weapon. This requires astute recognition, especially in the heat of a vicious fight. Fight positioning determines your tactical advantage. Optimally, a kravist will move quickly to a superior and dominant position relative to his opponent, known in krav maga parlance as the deadside. With the exception of the initial defensive movements against some impact weapon attacks, krav maga weapons defenses strive, when possible, to take the defender to the assailant's deadside which often provides a decisive tactical advantage. Once superior position and control of the weapon are achieved while simultaneously controlling the weapon to keep both you and bystanders safe, the assailant will have a minimal ability to defend or to counter your retzev counterattack. The defender's control of the weapon also keeps bystanders safe. Retzev, using all parts of your body seamlessly in coordinated concert, provides an overwhelming counterattack including, when necessary, turning the weapon on the assailant.

If both the defender and assailant are on the ground and the assailant decides in mid-fight to deploy a weapon, krav maga's weapon defenses on the ground are similar to its standing defenses. Movement on the ground is obviously different than when standing. Accordingly, the defenses must be modified. The nature of groundfighting can allow one opponent superior control and positioning, while the other opponent cannot run or evade as he might while standing. Again, krav maga groundwork against weapons is best defined as "what we do up, we do down" with additional specific groundfighting capabilities. We employ many of our standing combatives on the ground, including groin, eye, and throat strikes in combination with joint breaks and dislocations designed, if necessary, to maim your opponent.

the defender in the most advantageous position. We will examine this particular defense in detail in Figures 3.01 and 4.01. As noted, whenever possible, krav maga utilizes both a deflection-redirection combined with a body defense that moves the defender off the line of attack, or in the case of firearm disarms, out of the "line of fire." By deflecting-redirecting the incoming attack and simultaneously moving away from it combined with a counterattack, krav maga strives to create a fail-safe redundant defense. Not only is the attack thwarted by a deflection-redirection and simultaneous counterattacks, the defender is also not positioned where the assailant anticipated.

Analyzing the overhand edged-weapon attack example starts to put you in the mind-frame of a kravist skilled in weapons defenses. Let's go through this particular defense step-by-step (we will cover the technique in detail in Chapter 4). When facing deadly weapon assaults, such as an edged-weapon attack, krav maga provides the defender with the option of striking to vital areas such as the throat. Again, the immediate goal is to stop the assailant. This means neutralizing the assailant with soft tissue strikes and other combatives to then allow the defender to exert decisive control over the weapon.

One of Imi's more famous sayings was that you should be "so good that you do not have to kill." Imi also had another saying that some krav maga techniques were only useful to commandos or criminals. Of course, criminals have no place in krav maga. Therefore, some of krav maga's techniques are reserved for military and security teaching only.

Krav maga is flexible; instructors do not provide set instructions but, rather, a comprehensive blueprint. Learning by rote would violate krav maga's practicality and adaptability. However and wherever krav maga might be used, it must be used for the right reason—self-defense with the appropriate level of counterforce. An assailant armed with a weapon can clearly cause you serious bodily harm or kill you. Krav maga is both aggressive and decisive in countering weapon attacks. If you must physically engage the assailant, the goal is to deliver you from harm's way and dominate the assailant.

The law in most countries evaluates a person's response according to a "reasonable person standard." For self-defense, the operative language becomes "reasonable force." In other words, what would the reasonable person do, or how would he or she react, under the totality of the circumstances? Among the myriad facts involving a violent confrontation, the law analyzes a disparity in size and strength when adjudicating liability and criminal charges. When completing a weapon disarm against an assailant, if you control the weapon and the assailant is no longer a threat, you must cease your defensive actions. The moment you are deemed safe, any additional defensive actions may, in fact, become offensive actions.

If you continue to injure an assailant who is no longer a threat, you could face civil and criminal charges—especially if you deliberately turn the weapon on the assailant. For example, if you disarm a gunman and then shoot him repeatedly with his own weapon, you may be justified provided he kept coming at you. But, if you shoot him center mass and he goes down no longer presenting a threat, and you then walk up to him and shoot him point blank in the head—you have just executed someone and you will answer for it.

In short, to defend yourself, only use the amount of force commensurate with the threat. As tempting as it might be, to severely hurt or kill your assailant, you must make a deliberate conscious decision when to cease your counterattack. Granted, in the heat of the confrontation there is precious little or no time to weigh your options especially when reacting instinctively. Just remember, if the initial violent confrontation ends and you have time to contemplate your next move, the situation is no longer life threatening; do not continue your counterattacks. Disengage and wait for law enforcement officials to arrive or flee if necessary and then contact the authorities.

For armed law-enforcement personnel who have a sworn duty to protect the public, krav maga training teaches an officer to directly handle a threat coupled, importantly, with the ability to quickly de-escalate or escalate the appropriate level of force. Krav maga recognizes that when faced with a deadly threat, most officers will instinctively reach for a sidearm or, in a tactical situation, resort to a rifle/submachine gun (SMG). Therefore, krav maga teaches variations of the tactics incorporating streamlined weapon deployment and higher use-of-force options.

The Best Use of This Book

This book is designed for the novice and expert alike who would like to improve his or her chances of not just surviving an armed attack, but increasing the odds of prevailing against an armed attack without serious injury. Many students marvel that they can come to one krav maga class and regardless of their prior self-defense training, they walk away proficient—with a lasting knowledge—in the specific weapon disarms they just learned. For example, you could walk away from a single class taught by a qualified Israeli krav maga instructor and decisively disarm someone pointing a handgun at you or attacking you with an iron pipe.

The weapon defenses covered in this book assume you have no choice but to physically engage and defend. To be sure, in any situation involving an adversary with a weapon, the optimum solution would be to recognize the threat and steer clear of it. The best use of this book is to practice each technique as presented. You will find that each technique either builds upon a previous technique or complements a technique yet to be presented. You will find that the Israeli krav maga system relies on a few core movements that are highly adaptable to the myriad variables when confronting weapon removal and disarms.

Krav maga is designed to work for anyone regardless of athleticism, skill, size, or gender. Krav maga's popularity is in large part attributable to its practicality, simplicity, easy retention, and brutal effectiveness. We train groups of responsible civilians, law enforcement, and military personnel, all of whom have limited training time. We are able to teach them the proven techniques in this book in a condensed training period.

For example, one officer who had never taken any defensive tactics training beyond the basics he learned at his academy was skeptical toward krav maga's efficacy, took a six-hour handgun disarm seminar, and came away marveling at his newfound capabilities. In another large krav maga course I taught, a U.S. special forces operator, who later admitted to taking the course to disprove krav maga's methodology, also came away thoroughly convinced of the efficacy of krav maga's weapon disarms. He wondered why with his many years of top-tier training he had not been exposed to these simple yet formidable combat-oriented building blocks. Similarly, civilians with extensive martial arts background have also come away as krav maga converts, having learned that the same krav maga defense can be used to counter four different outside attacks to the head: a hook punch, an edged-weapon overhead stab, edged-weapon hook stab, or an edged-weapon slash.

Our krav maga trainees come away with a lasting knowledge to defend against weapon attacks that can be performed under stress. Of course, no book is a substitute for hands-on learning with a qualified Israeli krav maga expert instructor, but I hope to impart some of the more important principles and core tactics to hone your weapon defense skills. Most important, when locked in an armed confrontation, you must believe you will survive regardless of the injuries you might sustain in defending your life. There is a fine distinction between confident and over-confident. Do not mistake the latter for the former. If faced with a threat—not an imminent attack—if the circumstances do not favor disarming the assailant and you can comply or run away, do so.

Krav maga's evolution focuses only on street-proven tactics. If a technique should fail, Grandmaster Gidon either removes it or modifies it. Unlike other traditional self-defense systems, krav maga does not insist on implementing a particular strength, whether it is kicking, punching, or throwing, etc., to solve the problem. In other words, krav maga adapts to the nature and necessity of defending a particular weapon and family of related threats or attacks by relying on a few core weapon-oriented principles and tactics. Current Grandmaster Haim Gidon has modified several weapon defenses, which founder Imi Lichtenfeld formally approved in the mid-1990s. When applicable, these modified defenses are distinguished in the text from the first generation krav maga techniques.

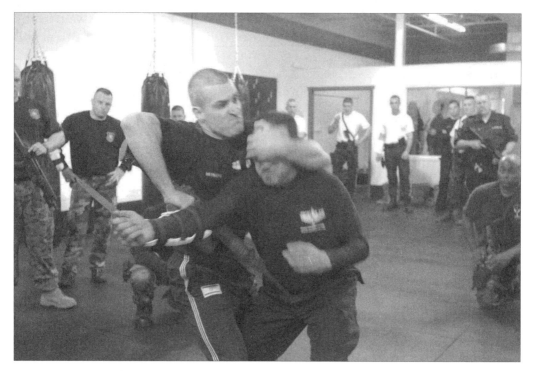

SWAT Training. Photo courtesy of Edward Greenblatt.

CHAPTER 1

Control Holds Reviewed

Prior to covering *krav maga* (means *contact combat* in Hebrew) weapon defenses, we need to revisit a few of krav maga's control holds, two of which are known as cavaliers. Cavaliers are designed to use your powerful hip muscle groups and bodyweight to torque an opponent's wrist to take him down while establishing strong control over the weapon for removal. There are three types of cavaliers frequently used in krav maga. Cavaliers are preceded by retzev combatives against the assailant, including full-force strikes to the groin, neck, eyes, and other vulnerable opportunistic targets. Control holds are used in krav maga to remove blunt and edged weapons and, sometimes, firearms from the assailant's grip.

Cavalier #1

This powerful takedown places enormous pressure on an opponent's wrist, forcing him down to the ground while placing strong control of the weapon. If necessary, you can follow up with a strong kick to the head, midsection, or groin along with an armbar or wristlock to remove the weapon.

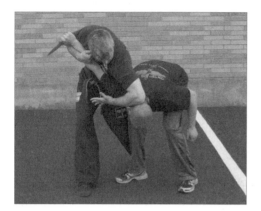

Figure 1.01a

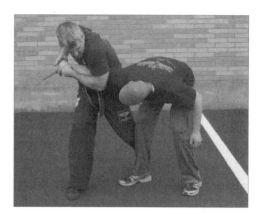

Figure 1.01b

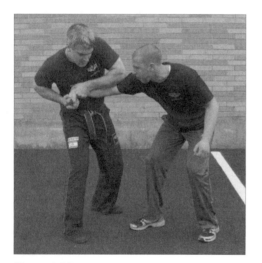

Figure 1.01c

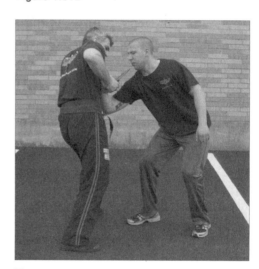

Figure 1.01d

Figures 1.01a–d. After administering combatives, for Cavalier #1, secure your opponent's right hand while you are positioned behind his right shoulder and to his side. If you are securing your opponent's right hand for the takedown, place your right hand on top of his right hand or "knuckles to knuckles." Your left hand then secures his right forearm just below the wrist. Do not grab the opponent's wrist because the grab hinders your desired objective of applying maximum torquing pressure to the wrist. Try to keep your elbows as close to your body as possible to best control the weapon and keep it away from you and directed toward the assailant.

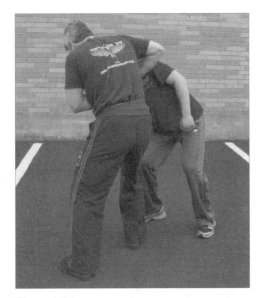

Figure 1.01e

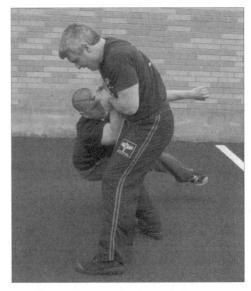

Figure 1.01f

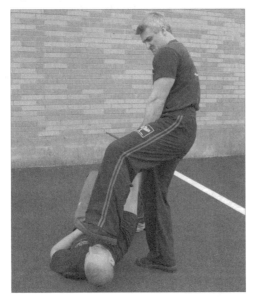

Figure 1.01g

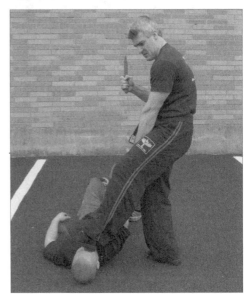

Figure 1.01h

Figures 1.01e–h. The wrist is flexible, but few people are flexible when applying simultaneous inward and side pressure. Think of the cavalier as driving your opponent's pointer finger toward his sameside shoulder. To apply the torquing pressure, as illustrated, take a one-hundred-eighty-degree rear step with your left leg (tsai-bake). If the opponent continues to present a threat, you may use a heel stomp to his head or body depending on your perception of his continued ability to resist.

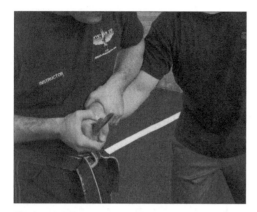

Figure 1.01i

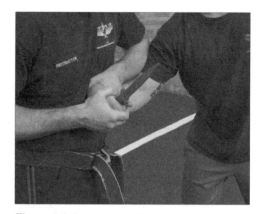

Figure 1.01j

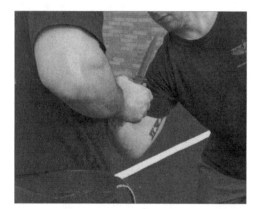

Figure 1.01k

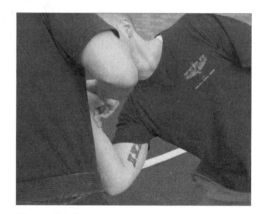

Figure 1.01l

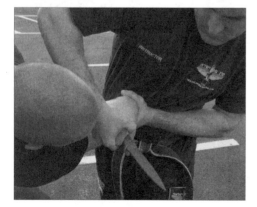

Figure 1.01m

Figures 1.01i–m. Close-up photos depicted of elbow and wrist control positioning. Note: A common mistake when controlling the weapon for the takedown is when the defender brings the edged weapon across his own throat or smashes a blunt weapon into his own head when applying the cavalier and removing the weapon from the assailant's grip. When you encounter a strong opponent, you may have to continue to "loosen him" up by using a knee strike, shin kick, or other combative, including a vertical uppercut elbow to the back of his clenched fist. These strikes both distract and physically undermine your opponent's ability to resist.

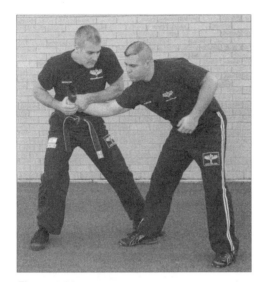

Figure 1.01n

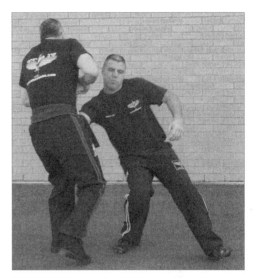

Figure 1.01o

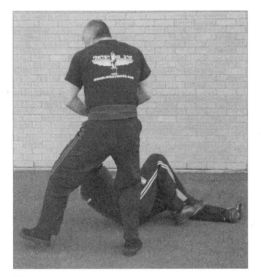

Figure 1.01p

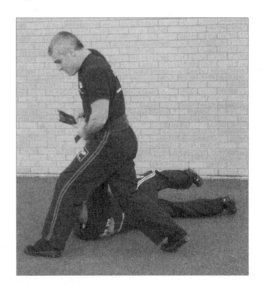

Figure 1.01q

Figures 1.01n–q. Your opponent may try to counter the technique by rolling out of the hold using his momentum. Once you have taken your one-hundred-eighty-degree (tsai-bake) rear step to take him off his feet, you can prevent his rolling by torquing his wrist in the opposite direction and pinning it to your thigh. Keep applying upward pressure to keep his right shoulder off the ground. Once you have taken your opponent down, do not let go of the wrist. Again, many offensive combatives can be used at this point, such as a heel stomp to the head, midsection or groin.

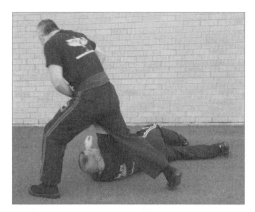

Figure 1.01r

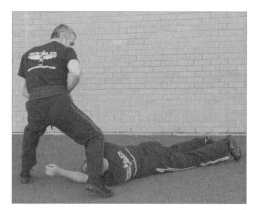

Figure 1.01s

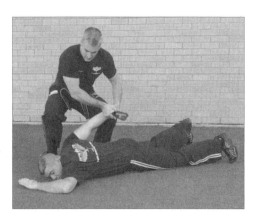

Figure 1.01t

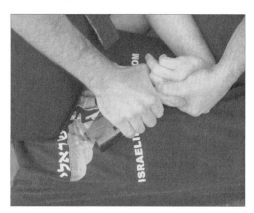

Figure 1.01u

Figures 1.01r–u. For law enforcement and security personnel, once you have taken the opponent down on his back, you may reverse him onto his stomach by yanking up on his arm and stepping one-hundred eighty degrees in the opposite direction while clipping arm just below the elbow with your knee to facilitate his turn. You are in strong position to collapse his straight arm for face down control of the weapon and the application of restraints. Figure 1.01v is a close-up depiction of the defender dropping his knees on the assailant's back and neck while placing pressure on the wrist to carefully pry the weapon free.

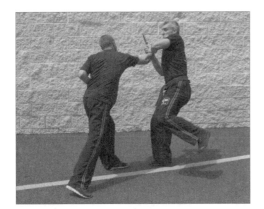

Figure 1.01v

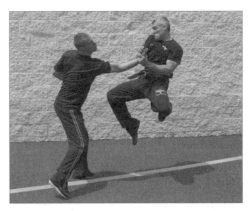

Figure 1.01w

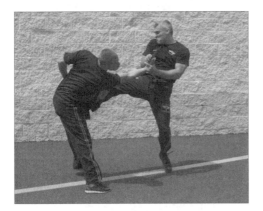

Figure 1.01x

Figures 1.01v–x. An advanced variation utilizes a jumping scissors kick to the opponent's groin while applying crushing wrist pressure to the opponent. To execute the kick properly, jump high on the kicking leg while pulling the non-kicking leg high into your chest to elevate the jump. (Both legs do not jump together.) Note: This disarming method with modification is used to take down an assailant threatening with a hand grenade.

Cavalier #2

Cavalier #2 is used when you have wrapped up the opponent's weapon arm from the inside such as when using an instinctive defense to defend an underhand edged-weapon attack. Rotate the assailant's hand to the inside by applying a joint lock to his shoulder and elbow. The Cavalier #2 wristlock involves moving from the inside control of the edged weapon-arm by trapping the assailant's arm across your chest.

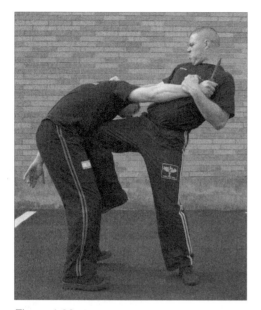

Figure 1.02a

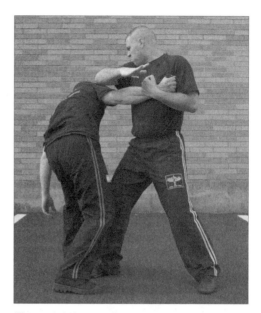

Figure 1.02b

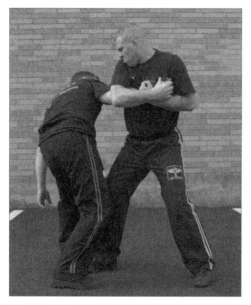

Figure 1.02c

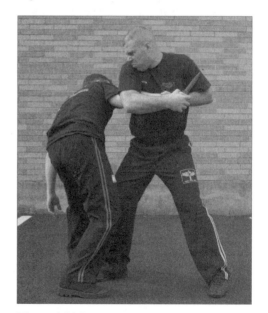

Figure 1.02d

Figures 1.02a–d. Once you have stopped the attack and sufficiently debilitated the assailant with combatives to establish firm control over his weapon arm, reach your hand across your chest to grab the back of the assailant's hand, placing the flat of your hand over the back of his hand. This movement creates a "knuckles to knuckles" position.

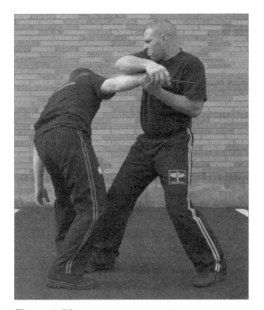

Figure 1.02e

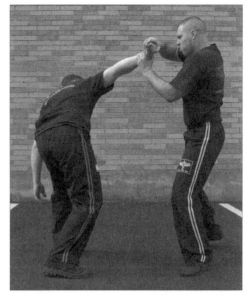

Figure 1.02f

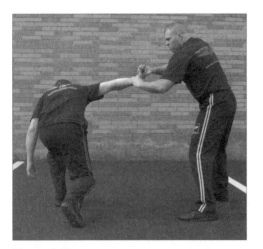

Figure 1.02g

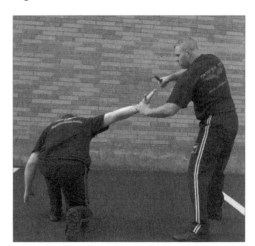

Figure 1.02h

Figures 1.02e–h. By positioning your knuckles down ("thumb to you") with your palm against the back flat side of his hand ("prayer" hold) with your opposite hand also facing down and parallel, rotate the assailant's hand down and away by taking a tsai-bake step. You know where the assailant's hand is positioned so you need not look at it. Keep your eyes on the assailant allowing you to pan for additional threats. A devastating finish to this technique is a sidekick to the assailant's nearside knee. Be sure to keep your elbows tight to your torso to maintain maximum control over the attacker's weapon arm and, when turning, keep the blade away from you. Do not bring the blade across your throat or face while rotating his arm.

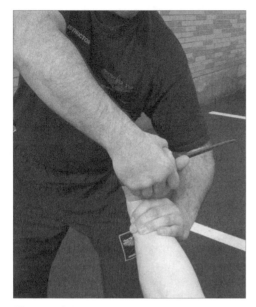

Figure 1.02i

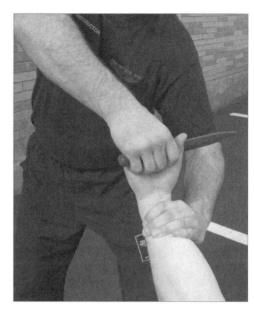

Figure 1.02j

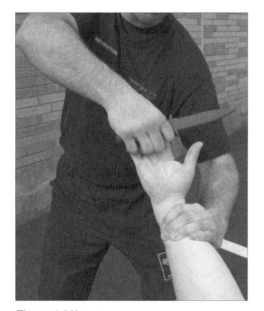

Figure 1.02k

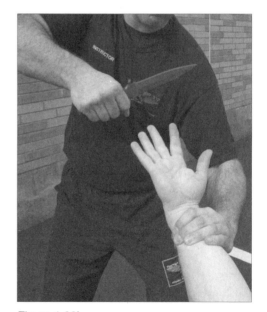

Figure 1.02l

Figures 1.02i–l. To remove the weapon from his grip, use the palm heel of your "knuckles to knuckles" hand to punch his wrist toward him using your hips and upper body in concert. For added power, you may momentarily release your grip to cock your arm slightly to palm heel through his wrist. As you break the wrist's posture, dig your fingers into his palm, wrapping around the weapon's grip. Use your fingers to strip the weapon and pry it from his grip.

Cavalier #3

Cavalier #3 is used when you have wrapped up the opponent's weapon arm from the inside and find it easier to keep the arm wrapped and trapped to apply a wristlock for weapon removal. Similar to Cavalier #2, the Cavalier #3 wristlock involves moving from inside control of the edged weapon arm by trapping the assailant's arm across your chest.

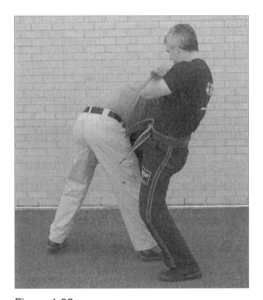

Figure 1.03a

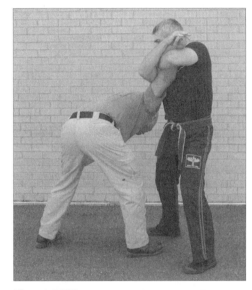

Figure 1.03b

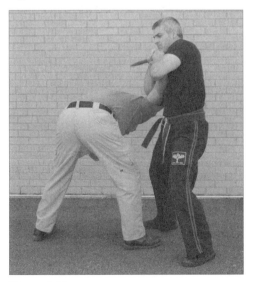

Figure 1.03c

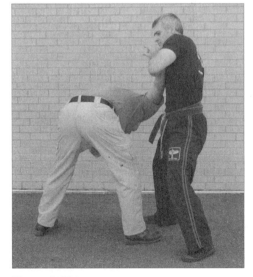

Figure 1.03d

Figures 1.03a–d. Caption on next page

Figures 1.03a–d. After you have stopped the attack and sufficiently debilitated the assailant with combatives to establish firm control over his weapon arm, reach your hand across your chest to grab the back of the assailant's triceps just above the elbow. Keep the weapon arm firmly in control across your chest. Rotate the assailant's arm, forcing the back of his weapon hand until it is parallel to the ground. Secure the weapon hand "knuckles to knuckles" and peel the hand down placing great pressure on his wrist. Be sure to keep additional pressure against his triceps with your elbow as you strip the edged weapon away. Note: To use Cavalier #3, the attacker must have an underhand grip—not an icepick type or overhand stab.

Control Hold A

This highly practical and effective control hold allows an assailant to be taken down face-first, swiftly with strong deadside positional control, and driven into the ground with dominant control over the weapon.

Control Hold A may also be applied with or without preceding retzev combatives. Again, usually in the case of a weapon, the defender has delivered strong preceding combatives and has control of the weapon arm before applying the specific hold. The hold places compliance or takedown pressure on the opponent's wrist and shoulder while controlling the weapon.

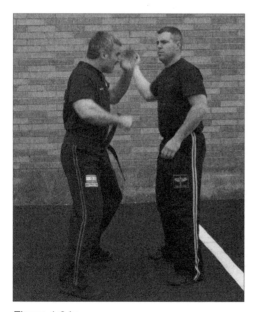

Figure 1.04a

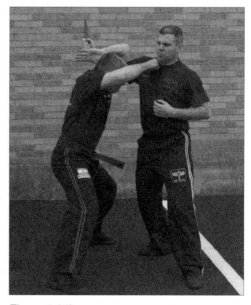

Figure 1.04b

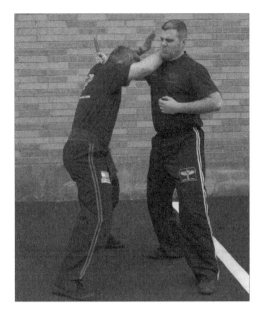

Figure 1.04c

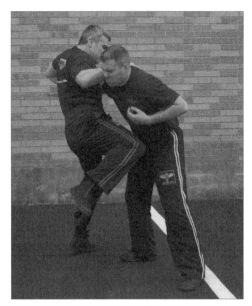

Figure 1.04d

Figures 1.04a–d. (Note: These photos depict a close slash that requires a modified block.) After administering combatives, if you are facing your opponent or the side of your opponent, grab his right wrist with your right hand. Another option is to grip the flat of the back of his hand by turning your wrist up to create pressure on his wrist. Raise your wrist up placing upward pressure so that his arm comes up with a ninety-degree bend with fingers toward the ground. Reach over the top of his targeted shoulder clamping down hard on the shoulder while snaking your right arm over the top of his targeted right arm across his shoulder to clasp your other arm.

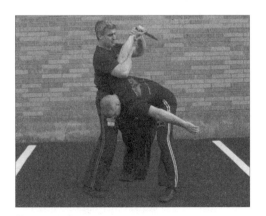

Figure 1.04e

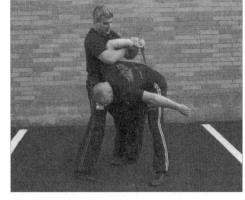

Figure 1.04f

Figures 1.04e–f. You must clamp down on the targeted shoulder to facilitate the lock. Reach around the arm and encircle it to grip your own forearm.

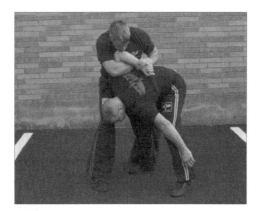

Figure 1.04g

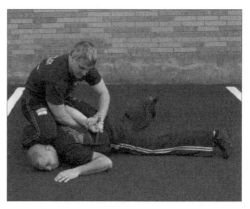

Figure 1.04h

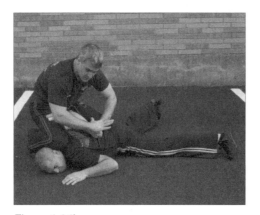

Figure 1.04i

Figures 1.04g–i. Bring his elbow and wrist close to your body, torquing the shoulder upward while keeping hard pressure on the shoulder. Note: By torquing the arm upward, an escape, especially using a scissors takedown or counter, becomes much more difficult. Take a one-hundred-eighty-degree (tsai-bake) step towards two o'clock with your right leg to bring down your opponent. As your opponent is going down, keep the grip tight. You may further secure him and the weapon by placing your right knee behind his elbow exerting pressure up on the shoulder and your left knee on top of his neck. To remove the weapon, peel the weapon from the assailant's grip using your thumb at the grip's base to keep the point directed at him and away from you.

Control Hold B

This highly adaptable control hold allows an assailant to be taken down swiftly backward with strong deadside control over an edged weapon.

Control Hold B may be applied with or without preceding retzev combatives. Usually in the case of a weapon, the defender has delivered strong preceding combatives and has control of the weapon arm before applying the specific hold. The hold places compliance or takedown pressure on the opponent's shoulder and wrist while controlling the weapon.

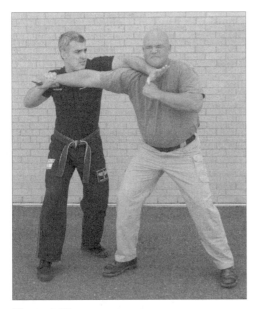

Figure 1.05a

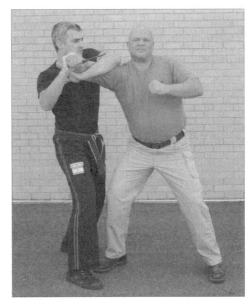

Figure 1.05b

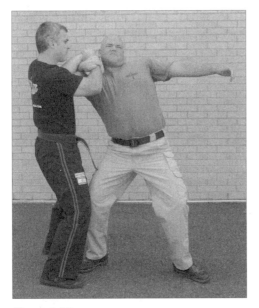

Figure 1.05c

Figures 1.05a–d. Caption on next page

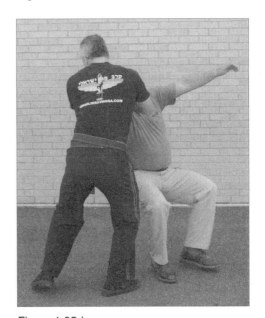

Figure 1.05d

Figures 1.05a–d. If you are facing or positioned to the side of your opponent, you must secure his right wrist with your left hand. Grip the flat of the back of his hand with a perpendicular grip. You can push his face away to cause a distraction. Curl his wrist in while slipping your other arm on the shoulder over the top of his targeted arm across his forearm using a Figure-Four grip. Then reach around the arm and encircle it to grip your own forearm tightening your right arm to your body. Bring his elbow and wrist close to your body; take a one-hundred-eighty-degree rear (tsai-bake) step with your left leg similar to Cavalier #1, bringing your opponent down. As your opponent is going down keep the grip tight. Once your opponent is down, you may use an additional knee strike to his head for further compliance or simply rest your knee on his head while exerting pressure on the wrist and shoulder. The opponent may also be rotated on his stomach.

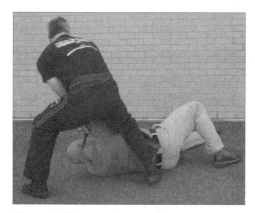

Figure 1.05e

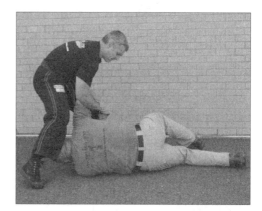

Figure 1.05f

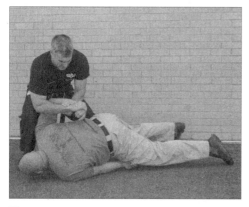

Figure 1.05g

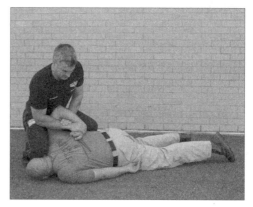

Figure 1.05h

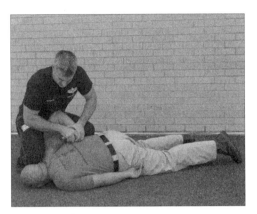

Figure 1.05i

Figures 1.05e–i. For law enforcement and security personnel or others who may wish to exert maximum control of the attacker, when effecting the hold against an unarmed or armed perpetrator, once you have taken the opponent down on his back, you may reverse him onto his stomach. Yank up on his arm while still maintaining your Figure-Four grip, then turn in the opposite direction. Do not break the movements by touching your knees to the ground. In this case, be sure not to collapse with him and keep upward pressure on his arm as you rotate him. Maintain the momentum of takedown into an immediate reversal onto his stomach. By keeping strong pressure on his wrist and shoulder to facilitate his turn, you have taken him down by combining a joint lock and a one-hundred-eighty-degree step in one direction. Take a one-hundred-eighty-degree (tsai-bake) step in the opposite direction, turning his wrist and shoulder in the opposite direction that you initially turned to take him down. To remove the weapon, peel the weapon from the assailant's grip using your thumb at the grip's base to keep the point directed at him and away from you.

You are in a strong position to remove the weapon, apply restraints, and control his movement.

Control Hold C

This highly practical and effective control hold variation also allows an assailant to be taken down immediately with strong deadside positional control while being driven face-first into the ground with dominant control over the weapon.

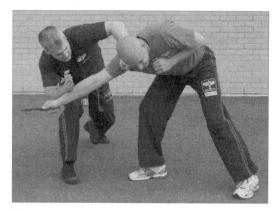

Figure 1.06a

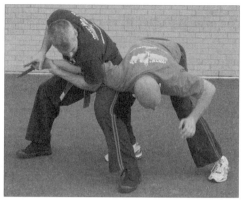

Figure 1.06b

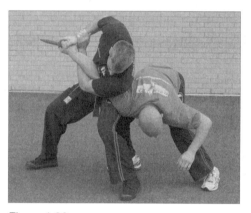

Figure 1.06c

Figures 1.06a–c. This control hold can be used when you have achieved dead-side position. Secure the assailant's wrist and use strong leverage to armbar the assailant to the ground. In addition, this control hold can be used as a strike to dislocate the assailant's elbow. You need to position yourself slightly behind and to the assailant's side. Assuming you are positioned to the assailant's right side, secure the assailant's right wrist with your right wrist. Pull his arm slightly outward and using your left forearm or ulna, exert strong pressure just above the assailant's right elbow while taking a left step and leaning your weight forward deep into his armpit. This will take the assailant face down to put you in a dominant control position. You can place a knee on his triceps to exert even greater compliance.

Face and Weapon Control Hold

Control of the assailant's head can work against any weapon; however, a handgun could be redirected at you, so you must be both diligent and careful to control the weapon as well.

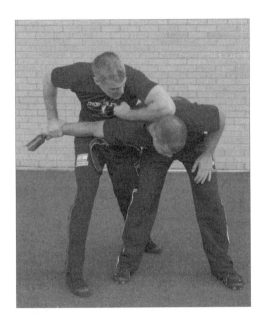

Figure 1.07a

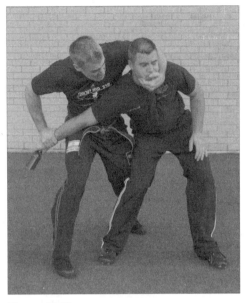

Figure 1.07b

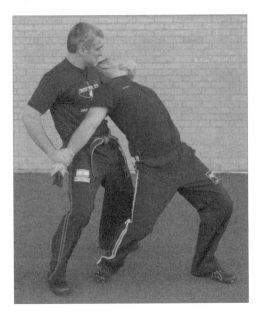

Figure 1.07c

Figures 1.07a–c. Controlling the assailant's head creates dominant control. Generally, if you control his head, you control his body. As with all weapon defenses, you must control the weapon and move to the assailant's deadside. Once you have achieved deadside position, reach around the assailant's head to secure his chin and head tight against your torso. Use your body combined with a one-hundred-eighty-degree (tsai-bake) step to take him down while maintaining strict control of the weapon.

Defense When the Handgun is Visible in the Front Waistband

An assailant could threaten you without deploying a handgun but by indicating or revealing its presence.

The defense resembles Frontal Handgun Defense #1. When you recognize the threat, react immediately.

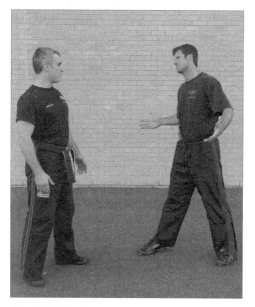

Figure 1.08a

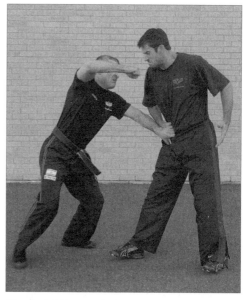

Figure 1.08b

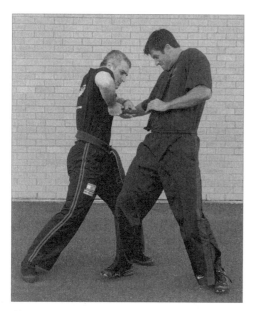

Figure 1.08c

Figures 1.8a–c. Decisively pin the handgun to the assailant's body controlling it at the rear of the slide while delivering multiple counterattacks. To remove the handgun, keep your weight pressed against the rear of the slide while sliding the handgun out and modify the removal process as learned in Frontal Handgun Defense #1. Note the importance of strong effective combatives to disable the assailant prior to removing the weapon.

Defense When the Handgun is in the Rear Waistband

You may be threatened by an assailant reaching behind his back to retrieve a firearm (or other weapon) from his rear waistband.

If the handgun (or anything else) is hidden in the rear of his waistband, one defensive option is to kick the would-be assailant in the groin and then close on him.

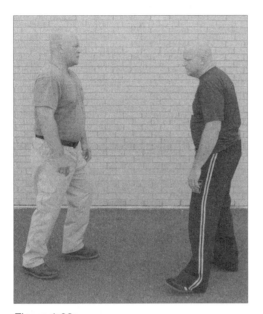

Figure 1.09a

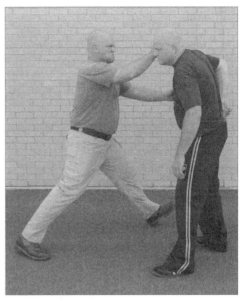

Figure 1.09b

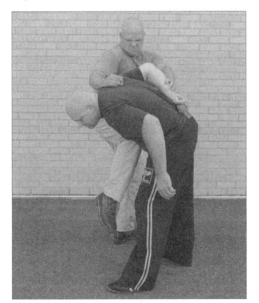

Figure 1.09c

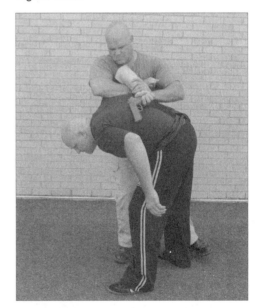

Figure 1.09d

Figures 1.9a–d. A second option (as depicted) is to close the distance with a knee strike to the groin or midsection while securing his reach arm with Control Hold B, a police hold often known as a kimura hold. You can also add a strong knee combative to take his level down.

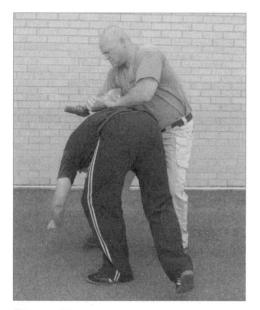

Figure 1.09e

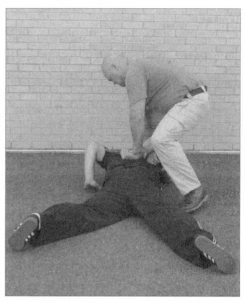

Figure 1.09f

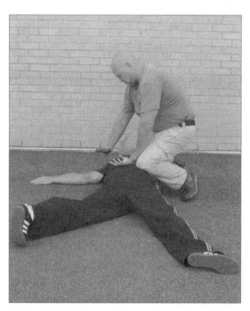

Figure 1.09g

Figures 1.9e–g. The advantage of the combined knee combative and control hold is just that: you debilitate the assailant while maintaining control over his weapon arm. To finish the hold and maintain control of the weapon, you need to transition from controlling his forearm to controlling his wrist and turn the opponent on his side to prevent him from using his free arm to retrieve the weapon.

Weapons of Opportunity

Before we begin to examine krav maga weapons defense techniques, it is helpful to review how a weapon of opportunity might enter a previously unarmed conflict. Not only must you be aware of a person's hands, body posture, and any pronounced threats, you must also be mindful of potential weapons of opportunity within his reach. For example, take a moment to look around you to improve your fighting chances. What could you immediately grab to use as a weapon or a distraction? Of course, your opponent could use the same object(s) as well. Remember, whatever you could use—so could an opponent. Anything and everything portable could possibly be used as either a weapon or a distraction. Here is a partial review list of how krav maga loosely groups weapons into the six categories:

1) Blunt objects. These include impact weapons, flashlights, stones, chairs, magazines, books, garbage can lids, briefcases, bottles, shoes, and wrenches.

2) Edged or point-like objects. These include broken bottles, keys, scissors, pens, forks, and cooking thermometers.

3) Flexible elongated objects. These include belts, chains, ropes, jackets, and towels.

4) Distraction objects and irritant liquids/sprays. These include keys, coins, watches, loose papers, cellular phones, jewelry, clothing, perfume, spittle, and aerosols. Note that certain liquids or sprays may result in a temporary or even more permanent blinding effect.

5) Defensive shield-type objects. These include chairs, briefcases, duffle bags, garbage lids and cans, car doors, and other shield-like objects.

6) Immovable environmental objects. These could include such varied things as using a curb to upend an assailant, racing around a parked car when being chased to then turn opportunely on the assailant, ramming an assailant's head into the ground, wall, or vehicle.

The following chapters show the most common weapon threats and attacks. There are any number of variations on these types of assaults and threats. Due to the number of photos that can be depicted, not every variation can be covered or mentioned. Neither can every technique can be shown in its entirety; however, the core weapon disarm-removal techniques are noted where applicable. Importantly, in some cases involving impact and edged-weapon defenses, after using a combative to disable the attacker, retreating, or escaping even when the weapon can be safely controlled or removed, may be the preferred option.

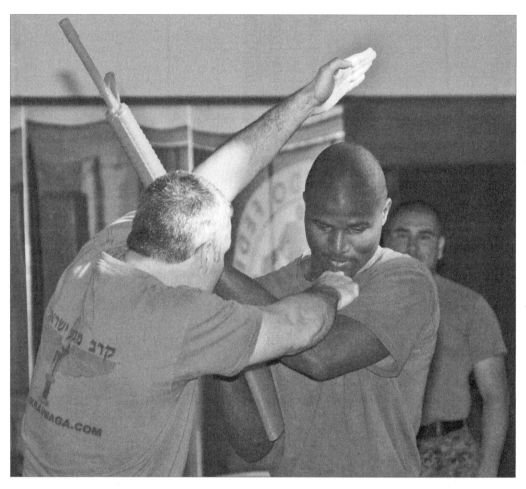

Training U.S. Marines. Photo courtesy of USMC Combat Camera.

CHAPTER 2
Impact-Weapon Defenses

Impact weapon attacks can come in many forms. For example, someone can try to smash you with a baton, hammer, crow-bar, bottle, chair, and anything onsite an assailant can pick up to use as a weapon. The three fundamental principles are either to (1) close the distance between you and the assailant while deflecting-redirecting the attack; (2) disengage until you recognize the correct timing to then close the distance; or (3) retreat straightaway. Obviously, for anything thrown at you, you need to make a body defense to make it miss. Attacks can come from myriad directions, heights, and angles in single swing attacks or multiple salvoes. Impact weapons (along with edged weapons) are often referred to in krav maga parlance as "cold weapons."

Recognize that a person with any type of blunt object in his hand could potentially use it as impact weapon or jettison it at you as a weapon or means of distraction. Notably, the end of the impact weapon generates the most force because the assailant's wrist is used as a fulcrum. Therefore, the most dangerous range of an attack is to be struck with the end of the weapon. In other words, the weapon's ballistic momentum decreases the closer you come to the assailant's swinging wrist. As noted, impact weapon defenses require the defender to stymie the attack by closing the distance to simultaneously deflect-redirect or absorb the swinging arm's (not the weapon's) impact. As with all krav maga defenses, the hand always leads the body to deflect-redirect in conjunction with simultaneous multiple counterattacks. Notably, impact weapons defenses—unlike edged and firearm defenses— move directly along the line of intended attack rather than "off the line" on which you will focus in Chapters 3–7.

We will focus on four common types of impact weapon attacks: overhead, overhead off angle, sideswing, and lower quadrant attacks. The danger, as with all weapon attacks, is that the assailant can change the angle of attack during the course of the attack to counter your initial defense. This situation is remedied by performing the same defense, regardless of the impact weapon's trajectory.

Overhand One-Handed Strike Defense

One of the most typical attacks with a blunt object is an overhead swing. In this technique, we assume the assailant is using his right hand and the defender is squared up to him or face-to-face. Execute the defense with your sameside (left) arm and a counterpunch with your right arm while controlling the weapon with your left arm.

Your goal is to close the distance to intercept and deflect-redirect the impact weapon harmlessly over your shoulder while delivering a simultaneous punch to the throat, jaw, or nose while trapping the weapon arm to remove the weapon from the assailant's grip while delivering more retzev combatives. As emphasized previously, the end of any impact weapon is the most dangerous as the momentum and velocity of the swing is at its greatest. One way to practice the deflecting-stabbing movement of the defense is to simulate diving into a pool with your arms in a "V" motion to pierce the water while keeping your legs straight. Keep the fingers together and simply touch both of your hands together at the fingertips resembling the inverted "V." Do not touch your palms together, only your fingertips, keeping your thumb pressed to the pointer finger (not exposed). Now, drop one arm into a straight punch position. Continue building this defense by aligning your deflecting-redirecting hand with a forward body lean, burying your chin into your shoulder. You could also use a pre-emptive straight kick to the attacker's groin or midsection to stop him, and then continue to press your counterattack.

The forward combat lean achieves two purposes: it both defeats the attack and protects your head. Essentially, you are diving/bursting into your assailant with the sameside arm and leg to close the distance while deflecting-redirecting the strike and simultaneously counterstriking. Another way to think about aligning your deflecting-redirecting arm is to stand in a neutral stance and jettison your arm directly out to meet an imaginary incoming attack. Proper arm alignment requires a slight curve in your hand that will intercept the attack. Keep the fingers together and the thumb attached to the hand; do not allow the thumb to stick out because of the danger in breaking it. The deflecting-stabbing defense, when timed correctly and with proper interception alignment, will redirect the object harmlessly along your arm over your head glancing off your back.

Once you feel comfortable with the initial defense, add a simultaneous punch with your other arm, thrusting both arms out together. Krav maga recommends a palm-down punch or keeping the palm of the hand parallel to the ground targeting the nose, chin, or throat.

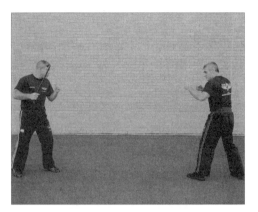

Figure 2.01a

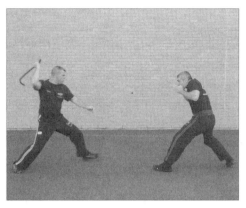

Figure 2.01b

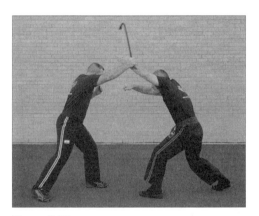

Figure 2.01c

Figures 2.01a–c. Time the defense and counterattack punch together. The next (literal) step forward is with your left leg closing the distance to the attacker. As you move into the assailant with your redirection and counterpunch, without breaking contact with the attacker's arm, loop your deflecting-stabbing arm over the assailant's impact weapon arm to secure the impact weapon arm.

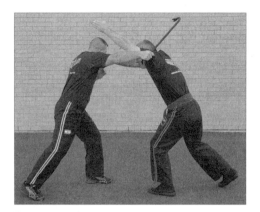

Figure 2.01d

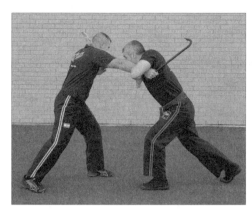

Figure 2.01e

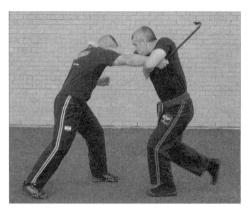

Figure 2.01f

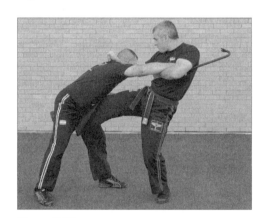

Figure 2.01g

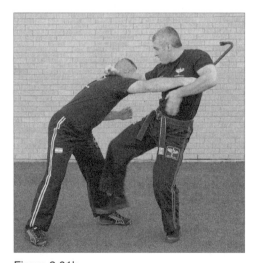

Figure 2.01h

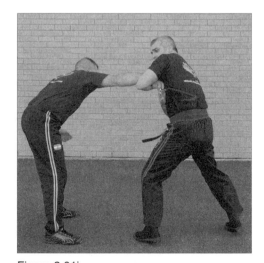

Figure 2.01i

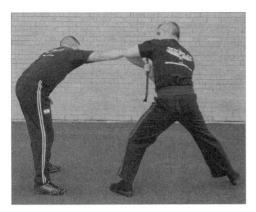

Figure 2.01j

Figures 2.01d–j. Continue your counterattack with a foreleg kick or multiple knee strikes to the groin depending on distance. The most popular method to remove the impact weapon is to use a one-hundred-eighty-degree step (tsai-bake) with your right foot to break or rip the impact weapon away from his hand without taking your eyes off the assailant. As you take your one-hundred-eighty-degree step, reach underneath with your right hand to rip the weapon away.

What to Do if the Assailant Drops the Weapon as You Counterattack

It is important to note that with all krav maga weapon defenses, your immediate strong counterattacks may force the assailant to drop the weapon. Of course, this removes you from the immediate danger of the weapon, but you must overcome any "tunnel vision" or "auditory exclusion"—a single focus on your assailant to the exclusion of everyone else. A second assailant could pick up the weapon to use it against you. Should the assailant drop the weapon, use whatever combatives and level of force you feel is necessary, but be sure to maintain awareness of where the weapon is. If you decide to confiscate the weapon, be aware of what onlookers might perceive, especially responding law enforcement or security personnel.

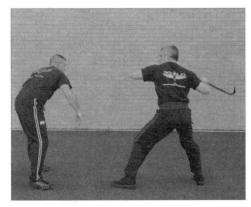

Figure 2.01k

Figures 2.01d–k. Continue your counterattack with a foreleg kick or multiple knee strikes to the groin depending on distance. The most popular method to remove the impact weapon is to use a one-hundred-eighty-degree step (tsai-bake) with your right foot to break or rip the impact weapon away from his hand without taking your eyes off the assailant. As you take your one-hundred-eighty-degree step, reach underneath with your right hand to rip the weapon away.

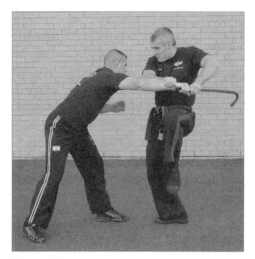

Figure 2.01l

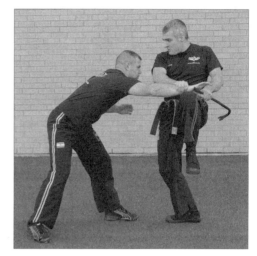

Figure 2.01m

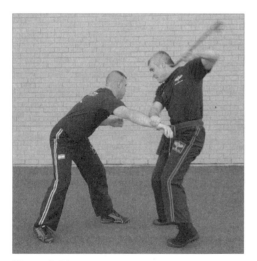

Figure 2.01n

Figures 2.01l–n. Another option after softening the assailant up with knee combatives is to switch control of the impact weapon from underneath your armpit to your left hand while using your right hand to grasp the assailant's forearm to then use your left knee to smash his hand while simultaneously yanking the impact weapon down and out. A final option to remove the impact weapon is to reach across your body with your free arm and grab the impact weapon using an inverted grip to sharply snap the impact weapon forcefully down and out of his hand. If necessary, with each impact-weapon removal technique, you can continue your counterattack with the impact weapon.

Overhand Defense Against a Long-Distance Attack or When Late

This defense is used when the attack comes too quickly or your defense is too late to close the distance to the attacker using a counterstrike punch.

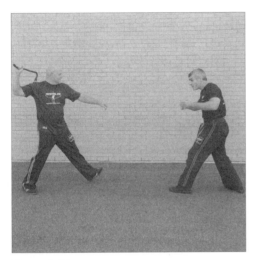

Figure 2.01o

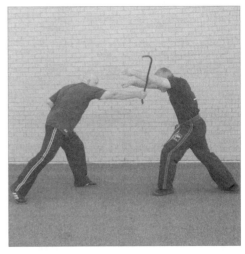

Figure 2.01p

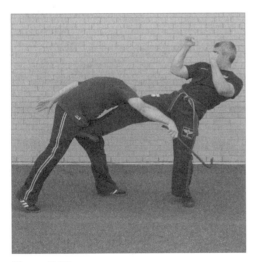

Figure 2.01q

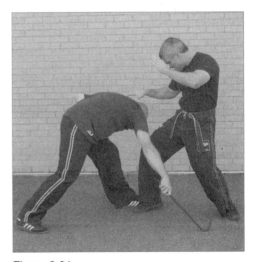

Figure 2.01r

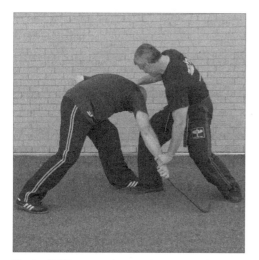

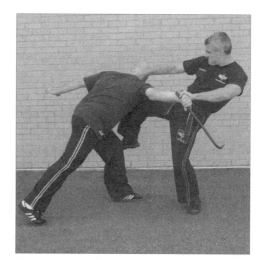

Figure 2.01s

Figure 2.01t

Figures 2.01o–t. As with your regular overhand defense, close the distance to deflect the incoming attack by stabbing your left arm while tucking your chin to intercept the incoming attack while delivering a simultaneous straight kick with the (right) opposite leg to the assailant's groin. The principles are the same as the previous technique. However, you may substitute a kick to the groin a millisecond after the deflection-redirection to allow you a longer-range counterattack to cover the distance between you and the assailant. Continue with combatives as necessary to neutralize the threat. Remove the impact weapon using one of the previous options.

Defending a One-Handed Overhand "Off-Angle" Defense

This attack comes indirectly or off angle, such as when the attacker is standing diagonal to you.

Similar to the direct overhand one-handed strike defense, you must align your nearside deflecting-stabbing hand with a forward body lean, burying the chin into your shoulder. The attack will again glide harmlessly along your arm and over your shoulder.

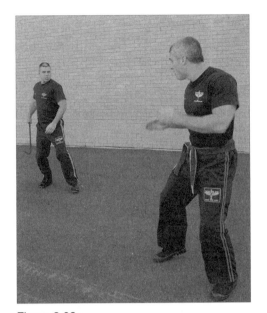

Figure 2.02a

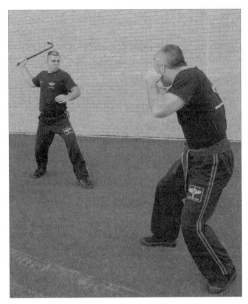

Figure 2.02b

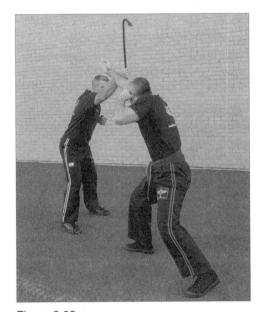

Figure 2.02c

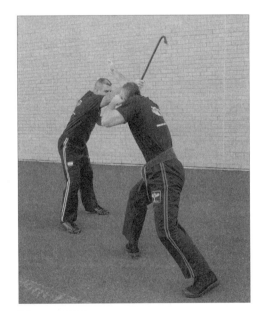

Figure 2.02d

Figures 2.02a–d. Step toward the assailant with the nearside leg and deflect with your nearside arm. As the impact weapon glides harmlessly overhead off your shoulder glancing off your back, take a forward step with your rear leg without breaking your deflecting-stabbing arm's contact with the assailant's arm.

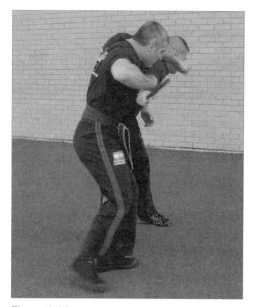

Figure 2.02e

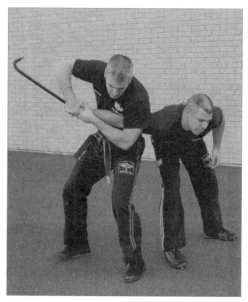

Figure 2.02f

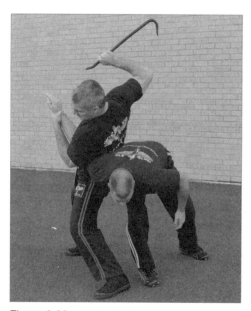

Figure 2.02g

Figures 2.02e–g. Turn your deflecting-stabbing arm's palm in and slide it down the assailant's arm maintaining contact until you reach the assailant's wrist to secure it against his body. Simultaneously, counterattack with a strong punch to the head. Continue your counterattack with multiple knee strikes to the assailant's nearside thigh or ribcage. To remove the impact weapon, the most popular option again, is to use a one-hundred-eighty-degree step (tsai-bake) with your right foot to break the impact weapon away from his hand without taking your eyes off the assailant. As learned in Figures 2.01j–m, after softening the assailant up with knee strikes to the groin, nearside thigh, or midsection to remove the impact weapon, switch control of the assailant's forearm to your left hand and grasp the impact weapon with your right hand. Keeping his elbow pinned to your midsection, forcibly rip the weapon away by stripping at the thumb. Apply an armbar by hyper-extending the elbow by positioning yourself deep into the attacker's armpit while you yank back on the arm.

As learned in Figures 2.01l–n, you could also use your right knee to smash his hand while simultaneously yanking the impact weapon down and out. If necessary, you can continue your counterattack with the impact weapon. A last option after you have secured the impact weapon and softened him with combatives is to use your free hand to reach around his head to execute a severe neck crank using a tsai-bake step to take him down as depicted in Figures 1.07a–c. Additional stomps may be used and the impact weapon can be removed using similar to the technique described above.

Defending a Two-Handed Overhead Chair or Stool-Type Attack

An assailant can attack with a double-handed overhead swing attack using a chair. The defense is similar to the one-handed overhead "off-angle" strike defense. The danger, as noted, is that the assailant can quickly change the angle of attack. As with the previous defense, this is remedied by performing the same defense regardless of the chair's trajectory.

Similar to the overhand one-handed strike defense, close the distance to deflect by aligning your deflecting-stabbing hand with a forward body lean, burying the chin into your shoulder.

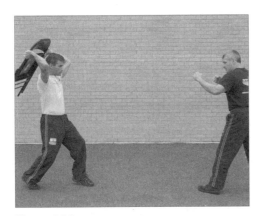

Figure 2.03a

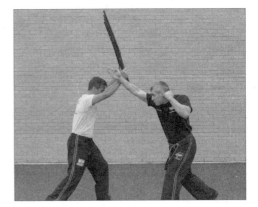

Figure 2.03b

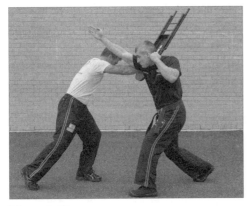

Figure 2.03c

Figures 2.03a–c. Burst toward the assailant with the opposite leg as your deflecting-stabbing arm. Your slightly bent hand will intersect just above the assailant's nearside hand holding the chair or stool. While the overhead chair attack glides harmlessly overhead, take a forward step with your rear leg without breaking your deflecting-stabbing arm's contact with the assailant's arm. The attack will again glide harmlessly along your arm over your shoulder and glance off your back.

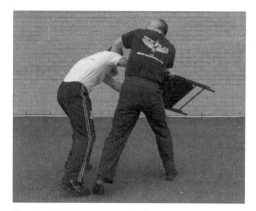

Figure 2.03d

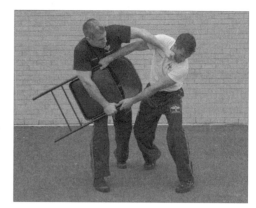

Figure 2.03e

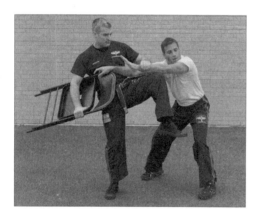

Figure 2.03f

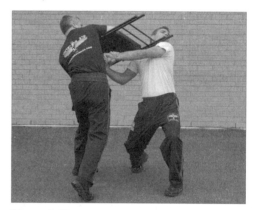

Figure 2.03g

Figures 2.03d–g. Turn your deflecting-stabbing arm's palm in and snake it around the assailant's arm(s) while counterattacking with strong punches or over-the-top elbow strikes with your free arm combined with knee strikes. Depending on the width of the chair and your arm length, you may not be able to ensnare the assailant's both arms. In this case, you must control his nearside arm by transitioning your deflecting-stabbing arm into a tight overhand grip. Note: Be careful the assailant does not release his nearside arm to control the chair with his farside arm, which could then be used to attack you with a "hook" or "whip" type of attack or a backhanded attack. If necessary, as you initiate combatives, kick the chair away. Note that kicking the chair away does not necessarily violate krav maga's cardinal principle of always controlling the weapon. By kicking the chair away, you are controlling the weapon by the only means at your disposal. If another assailant picks up the chair to resume an attack on you, krav maga uses control techniques to put your first assailant in the line of fire. In a worst-case scenario, you will have to defend against a second attack. Of course, you can disable the assailant who may drop the chair allowing you to pick it up, and, if necessary, use it as a cold weapon.

Defending a Two-Handed Overhead Swing Attack

An assailant can attack with a double-handed overhead swing attack. The defense is similar to the one- handed overhead "off-angle" strike defense. The danger is that the assailant can change the angle of attack. This is remedied by performing the same defense, regardless of the impact weapon's trajectory. See Figures 2.03a–g photos for the over-the-head chair defense to remove the weapon or you may use the tsai-bake weapon removal method as depicted in Figures 2.02e–g.

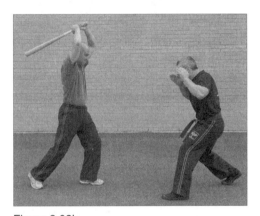

Figure 2.03h

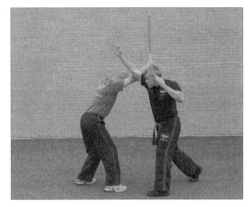

Figure 2.03i

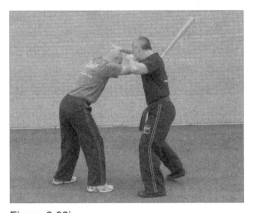

Figure 2.03j

Figures 2.03h–j. Similar to the direct one-handed overhead strike defense, you must close the distance to deflect-re-direct the incoming impact weapon by aligning your deflecting-stabbing hand with a forward body lean while burying the chin into your shoulder. Step toward the assailant with the opposite leg as your deflecting-stabbing arm. The attack will again glide harmlessly along your arm over your shoulder glancing off your back. As the two-handed overhead attack glides harmlessly overhead, take a small forward step with your rear leg without breaking your deflecting-stabbing arm's contact with the assailant's arm. Turn your deflecting-stabbing arm's palm in and snake it around both of the assailant's arms while counterattacking with strong punches or over-the-top elbow strikes with your free arm combined with lower body combatives.

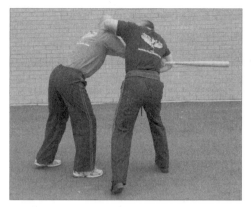

Figure 2.03k

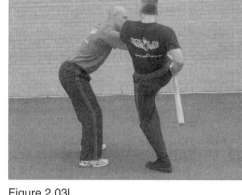

Figure 2.03l

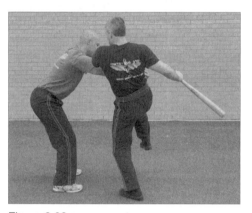

Figure 2.03m

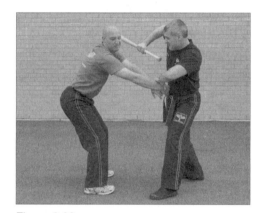

Figure 2.03n

Figures 2.03k–n. You may remove the weapon as described for previous techniques (Figures 2.01m–o and 2.03e–g) to press the counterattack, using it and other combatives. The only difference is you are ripping the weapon away from two hands instead of one. Another option is to deflect and continue a one-hundred-eighty-degree (tsai-bake) step movement after your second step with your rear leg to allow strong control over the arms and the ability to reach around the assailant's head with your free hand to use a neck crank to take him forcefully down with a tsai-bake step. You can then stomp him for good measure and break away the impact weapon using your preferred method. Lastly, an armbar is also available, if you have secured the attacker's arms above the elbows to facilitate removal of the impact weapon.

Defending a Sideswing Impact-Weapon Attack

Note that Israeli krav maga founder Imi Lichtenfeld approved of Grandmaster Haim Gidon's modification to the first generation defense, which had previously involved closing the distance by placing your nearside hand against your nearside thigh and bringing up your farside hand to protect your face. The tactic is to burst into the assailant and secure the control of the impact weapon. This defense is less preferred because an assailant can easily change the angle of attack to penetrate the hand protecting the head or swing low to attack the knees.

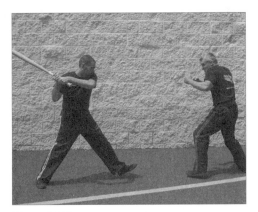

Figure 2.04a

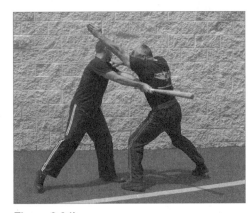

Figure 2.04b

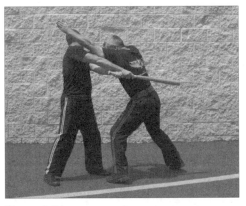

Figure 2.04c

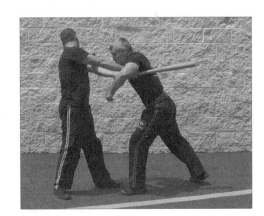

Figure 2.04d

Figures 2.04a–d. With your arm positioned to deflect an overhead attack, burst inside the attack arc to absorb the impact of the assailant's arms with your lateral muscle while delivering a simultaneous punch.

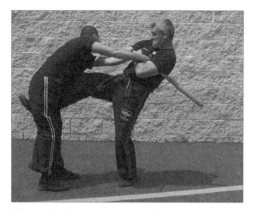

Figure 2.04e

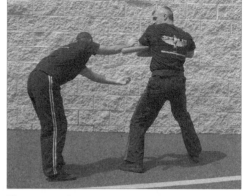

Figure 2.04f

Figures 2.04e–f. Secure the impact weapon as you would against a one-handed midsection attack adjusting as necessary, and press your counterattacks and weapon removal as previously learned. Again, the great advantage of this defense is that you can defend against an overhead or sideswing attack even if the assailant used a feint signaling he would attack one way, but changed the angle and direction of the impact weapon mid-attack. This defense is also used against a backhanded sideswing attack by deflecting-stabbing with your outside arm and punching with your inside arm.

Defending a Low Sideswing Impact-Weapon Attack

An assailant might try to attack your legs with a low swing.

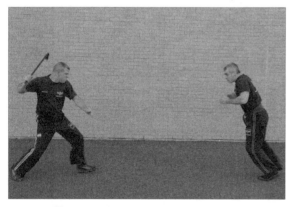

Figure 2.04g

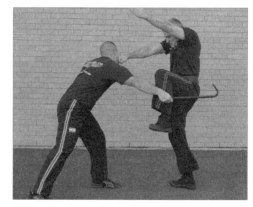

Figure 2.04h

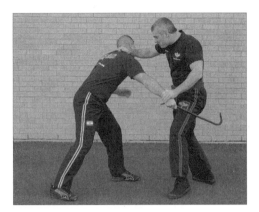

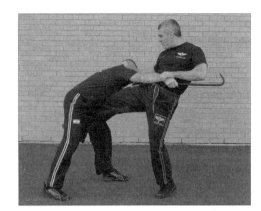

Figure 2.04i   Figure 2.04j

Figures 2.04g–j. The krav maga defense against an assailant swinging low at your legs is similar to the defense used against a low roundhouse kick. You will add a "bursting inside" movement to close the distance with the overhead defense combined with a simultaneous punch counterattack. Contact is made with your nearside leg's shinbone to the assailant's forearm. Your upper body is positioned as you would defend against an overhead attack. Use retzev to press the counterattack because this defense does not provide immediate control of the assailant's arm. After disabling the attacker, you can control the weapon arm by gripping the forearm or looping your sameside arm around the weapon arm while continuing to close the distance with simultaneous combatives. Remove the weapon as learned in Figures 2.01i–k or 2.01l–n.

Note: If the assailant were to swing from low to high (similar to a forehand swing of a tennis racket), you would use the same defense as a low sideswing attack to ensure defending at any angle.

Defending an Attacker Using Two Impact Weapons

Defending against two impact weapons is difficult and requires superb timing. As with the krav maga's other weapon defenses, close the distance to neutralize the weapon and counterattack.

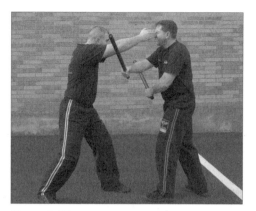

Figure 2.05a

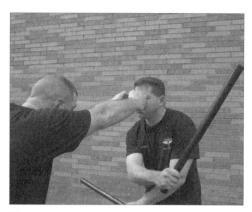

Figure 2.05b

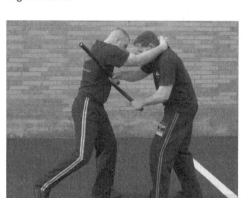

Figure 2.05c

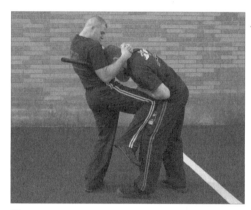

Figure 2.05d

Figures 2.05a–d. Defending against an attacker who is using two edged weapons inter-changeably or alternating his swings is challenging. With correct timing, you can defend as you normally would against one weapon moving on the centerline or you can attempt to move to his deadside. However, against a skilled opponent, moving to his deadside can be extremely difficult because he can simply pivot away from you and continue his attack. Another strong option, as depicted, is to burst into him using a diving motion with both hands affording protection with both arms. In other words, you are pointing both of your hands inward rather than one inward with the opposite delivering a punch. Once you close against the attacker, immediately try to clinch him against his torso by wrapping your hands around the back of his head (not the base of his skull) to pin his hands. Deliver debilitating knee combatives.

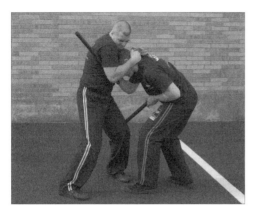

Figure 2.05e

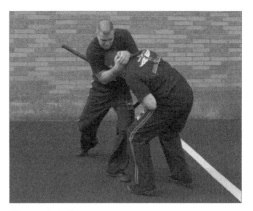

Figure 2.05f

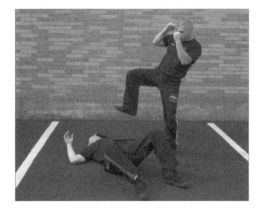

Figure 2.05g

Figures 2.05e–g. From a strong clinch, if you have not dropped your attacker with your knee combatives, you can take your attacker down by pulling his head into your chest and sharply turning his head using a one-hundred-eighty-degree pivot (tsai-bake) step. Use heel stomps to neutralize any continued threat.

Defending a Chain or Whip-like Attack

Defending against a chain or whip-like attack requires superb timing. As with the krav maga's other weapon defenses, close the distance to neutralize the weapon and counterattack.

To defend against a twirling attack while using correct timing, drop your level to come under the weapon's arc either using the preferred method, a roll into a takedown or, alternatively, a two-legged tackle.

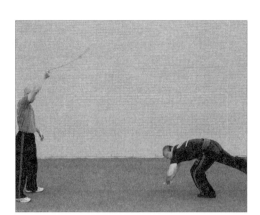

Figure 2.06a

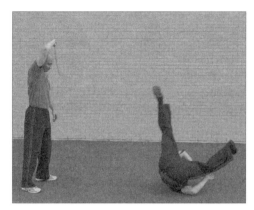

Figure 2.06b

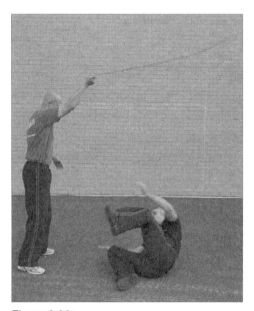

Figure 2.06c

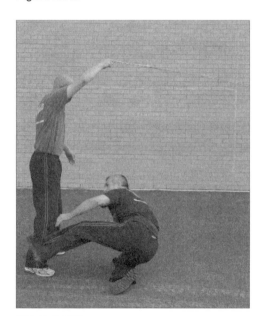

Figure 2.06d

Figures 2.06a–d. For the roll, you must judge your distance correctly. Roll properly by curling your body into a tight ball and burst into the assailant.

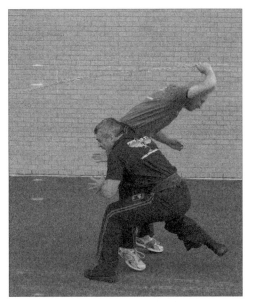
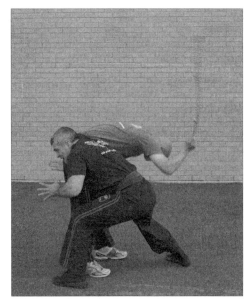

Figure 2.06e

Figure 2.06f

Figures 2.06e–f. Deliver a forearm strike in between his legs to his groin.

Another option is to slide in on your side (similar to sliding into a baseball diamond base) with a sidekick to the knee while covering your head. On concrete or other rough ground, the slide could be both painful and difficult. Sliding on a smooth training floor is very different from sliding on concrete, which creates decidedly more friction, shortening your ability to slide while also creating great discomfort.

Defending an Overhead Impact Attack When on the Ground

These modifications to the defenses you have already learned are designed as a last resort if you find yourself with your back to the ground and an assailant standing over you with an impact weapon.

It is difficult to use the previous arm defenses against an overhead impact attack because you are on your back. Bursting in to intercept the attack is not possible. Your legs become your best options. Of course, you can kick the assailant's legs to preempt his ability to attack you in addition to the depicted leg deflection defense.

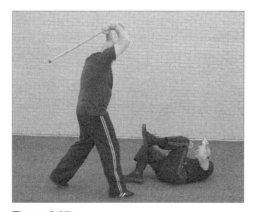

Figure 2.07a

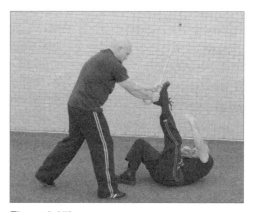

Figure 2.07b

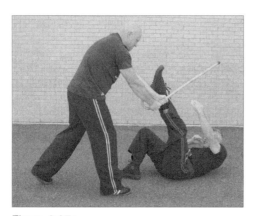

Figure 2.07c

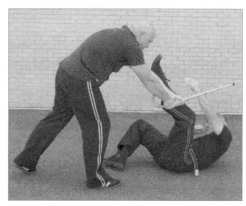

Figure 2.07d

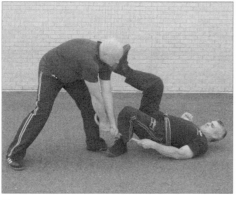

Figure 2.07e

Figures 2.07a–e. Use the nearside leg to intercept the incoming attack by using your foot to meet the attacker's hand. If the timing is correct, the impact weapon will glide harmlessly off your foreleg while you can use your other leg to kick the attacker in the groin, midsection, or head. Be sure to cover up with your arms in case the weapon continues descending toward your head.

Defending an Upward Rifle-Butt Stroke

A typical cold-weapon rifle combative is an uppercut strike. The defense is similar to defending against a straight punch, uppercut punch, or straight stab.

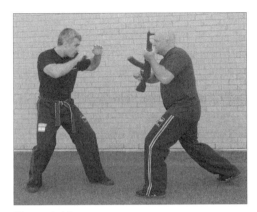

Figure 2.08a

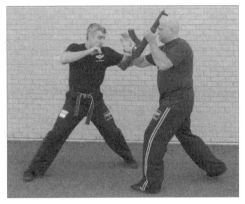

Figure 2.08b

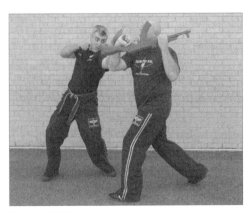

Figure 2.08c

Figures 2.08a–c. From your regular left outlet stance, your left arm leads the body to parry the rifle butt. The arm should be bent approximately to a seventy degree angle to deflect-redirect the assailant's upward rifle butt attack while making a subtle sidestep to the left. The parrying movement is no more than four- to six-inches and leads the body's defensive movement—as with most krav maga defensive tactics. This deflection-redirection is not an uncontrolled swipe or grab at the assailant's incoming arm (a common mistake when first learning the technique). The defensive arm makes use of the entire length of the forearm or from the pinky to the elbow to deflect any change in the height of the opponent's stab attempt. The movement rotates the wrist outward so that your left thumb, kept attached to the hand with all fingers pointing up, turns away from you as contact is made with the opponent's arm to redirect the incoming thrust. After the parry is made and without breaking contact with the assailant's arm, hook the assailant's arm by cupping your left hand, wrapping your left thumb around his forearm for control, and pinning the arm against the assailant's torso while delivering debilitating counterpunches to the throat or jaw.

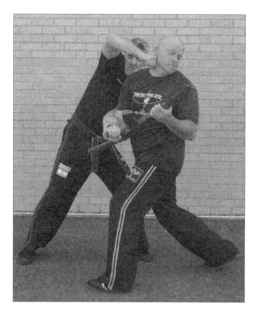

Figure 2.08d

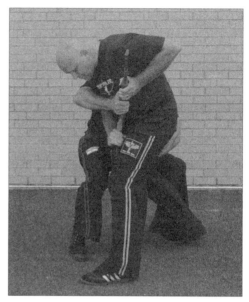

Figure 2.08e

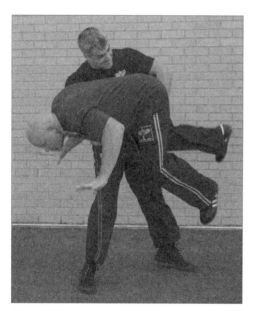

Figure 2.08f

Figures 2.08d–f. After you strike the assailant several times, transition your non-attacking arm to control the rifle. As you transition, sink your hips and thrust your other arm through the assailant's legs in order to first strike and then grab his groin. Load your hips properly by bending your knees with your back straight. Clutch the assailant's groin and pick him up to "bucket dump" him face-down. Once you dump him face-first, continue with any additional combatives, such as heel stomps or taking his back while administering punches or elbows to the back of his head or neck. To remove the weapon, either slide it out from beneath him or turn his right shoulder toward you to keep the muzzle pointed into the ground.

Defending a Horizontal Rifle-Butt Stroke

A typical cold-weapon rifle combative is a horizontal strike. The defense is similar to defending against a horizontal elbow strike.

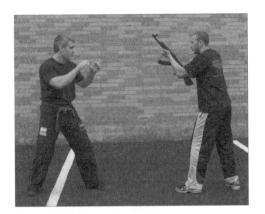

Figure 2.09a

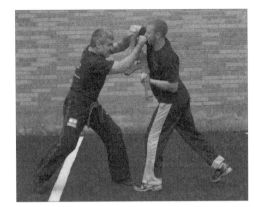

Figure 2.09b

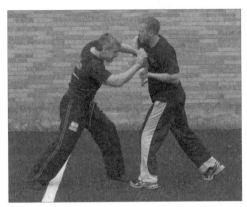

Figure 2.09c

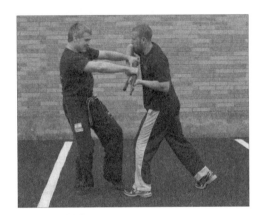

Figure 2.09d

Figures 2.09a–d. To defend against this powerful strike, you must block with the fleshy underside of your arms flexed at approximately a seventy-degree angle. Deliver a simultaneous shin kick or knee to the groin while bracing against the strike. As you deliver the strike, secure the weapon and invert inward to forcing the magazine into the assailant.

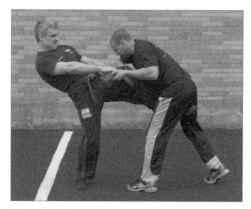

Figure 2.09e

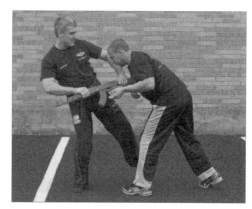

Figure 2.09f

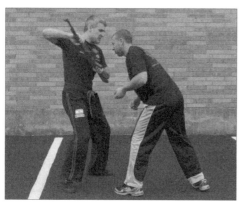

Figure 2.09g

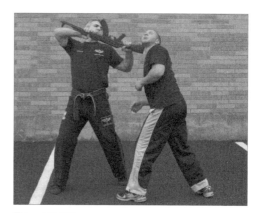

Figure 2.09h

Figures 2.09e–h. Remove the weapon and deliver additional cold weapon combatives as necessary.

Defending an Impact-Weapon Front Choke

An attacker may try to choke or crush your windpipe with an impact weapon.

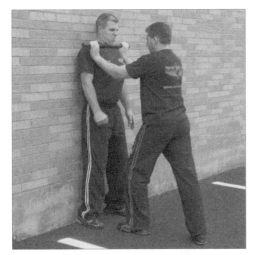

Figure 2.10a

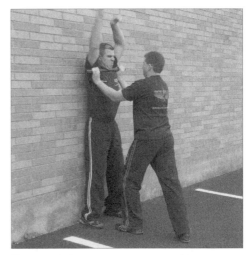

Figure 2.10b

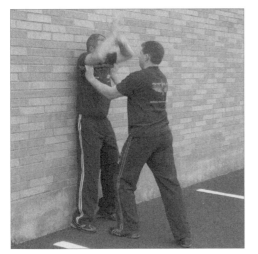

Figure 2.10c

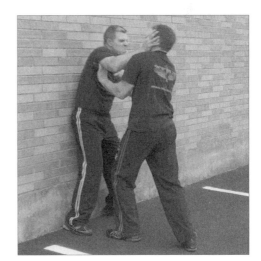

Figure 2.10d

Figures 2.10a–d. The defense, as with all krav maga choke defenses, is to tuck your chin and remove the threat with a simultaneous decisive counterattack. To clear and remove the threat, raise your arms above your head and bring them sharply down to force the choking implement to your chest. Immediately use both hands for eye gouges followed by retzev. The same defensive tactic would be used if your back were to the ground and the assailant on top of you combined with a hip buck release or to the side and pressing down on your throat with an elongated weapon.

Defending a Pulling Impact-Weapon Rear Choke

An attacker may try to choke or crush your windpipe with an impact weapon from behind you.

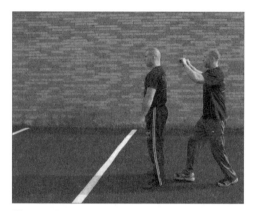

Figure 2.11a

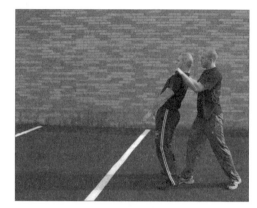

Figure 2.11b

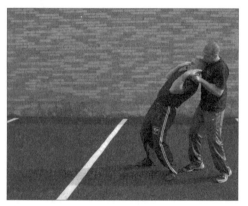

Figure 2.11c

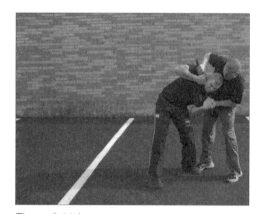

Figure 2.11d

Figures 2.11a–d. The defense against an attacker choking with an impact weapon from the rear using a pull is a modification of krav maga's basic forearm choke defense from the rear. The defense depicted involves a simple direct turn while securing the choking implement with both arms and yanking down with your core to alleviate pressure against your throat. On detection, turn your head to one side to protect your windpipe and turn inside (to the side you have turned your jaw) toward the assailant to harness both your momentum and his momentum. Maintaining a strong grip while pinning the weapon to your chest, continue to turn into the attacker to deliver knee strikes.

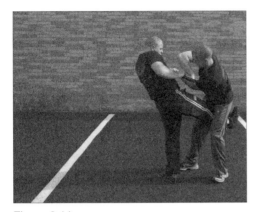

Figure 2.11e

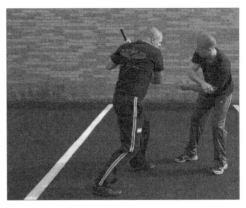

Figure 2.11f

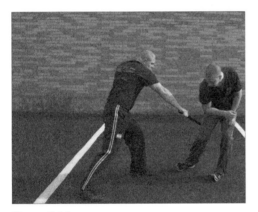

Figure 2.11g

Figures 2.11e–g. As you turn forcefully, you will likely cross his arms facilitating the weapon's removal by continuing to twist it combined with knee combatives. As you turn, simultaneously deliver a knee strike to the groin. Release the weapon and use it as necessary. Continue to counterattack using knee combatives and any other strikes as opportune.

An alternative defense, similar to the previous defense, is to tuck your chin, turning directly into the assailant.

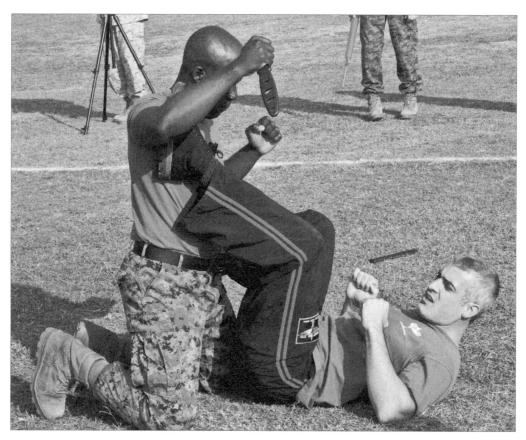

Training U.S. Marines. Photo courtesy of USMC Combat Camera.

CHAPTER 3

Leg Defenses Against Edged-Weapon Attacks

Edged-Weapons Introduction

You will need any and every advantage to defend against a determined assailant using an edged weapon. An edged weapon does not jam or run out of ammunition and can seriously injure you with every thrust or slash. A significant number of the population worldwide carries folding edged weapons or some other type of cutting instrument. Kitchen knives are accessible to just about anyone bent on doing harm. Never underestimate the harm an amateur but determined attacker can inflict—let alone someone skilled in edged-weapons use. Essentially, anyone with an edged weapon in his or her hand could be a deadly threat, particularly if he or she has no compunction about getting up close and personal.

Slashing to the jugular and major arteries is usually fatal, but lacerations to the other parts of the body are generally not. Thrusting wounds are far more dangerous. Puncture wounds of more than 1.2 inches can produce instant shock and seriously damage or shut down internal organs. When defending against a resolute attacker using an edged weapon, it is likely that you will be wounded. Of course, try to prevent wounds to your eyes, neck, torso, and major arteries. Nevertheless, whatever injuries you might sustain, relentlessly pursue your defense and counterattacks to end the threat. In short, the longer duration of the edged-weapon attack, the less likely you are to survive it. Once you successfully defended and neutralized the attack, immediately check yourself for wounds. You must immediately think about triage. Seek professional help right away, and if unavailable, administer self-triage.

Running away from an edged-weapon threat is, perhaps, the best option. If you must engage the assailant, krav maga once again emphasizes simultaneous defense and counterattack. The counterattacks must be targeted and forceful. The goal in striking an attacker's eyes, nose, windpipe, groin, and knees is to short-circuit his ability to continue the attack. Damage the attacker as much as possible to destroy both his physical ability and mental resolve to continue the attack. Attempting an edged-weapon disarm without debilitating counterattacks can, and will, get you seriously hurt or killed. While krav maga emphasizes simultaneous counterattacks and weapon control as soon as possible, you may have to counterattack and then disengage only to counterattack again. This must occur only when you deem it safe to close the distance, hurt the attacker, control the attacker, and remove the weapon.

Judging distances, the logical progression of a weapon's attack path(s) even when initially blocked or redirected, and the varied angles of attack are paramount to a successful defense. My good friend, Sgt. Major Nir Maman (res.), one of the lead krav maga instructors for the Israel Defense Forces Special Operations School, says it best: "If your assailant deploys an edged weapon, your best response is to make yourself disappear. If you cannot disappear, your next best response is to pull out a firearm. If you do not have a firearm available, you want a long-range impact weapon such as a lead pipe where you can batter his edged-weapon hand while staying out of range of the edged weapon." Nir's obvious point is how dangerous an edged weapon can be. Edged weapons are often referred to in krav maga parlance as "cold weapons."

Israeli krav maga uses two ranges in combination with body defenses to defend edged-weapons attacks: legs or hands. Either type of defense usually takes the defender off the line of attack in a position to deliver strong-counterattacks, with one exception: the instinctive defense against a surprise underhand attack. With krav maga hand defenses, employ a block or deflection-redirection when possible, with a body defense, combined with effective simultaneous counterstrikes, preferably to the assailant's throat, groin, or eyes.

Kicks are usually employed when the defender sees the edged weapon at long range. Kicks harness your most powerful muscle groups and have the longest range of any of your personal weapons. In addition, kicks can be combined using shield-like objects, such as a bag or briefcase, to simultaneously block or deflect-redirect an edged-weapon attack away while delivering a debilitating combative to the assailant's groin or knee. Strong defensive kicks with glicha keep the edged weapon farther away from you and are also best to stop a charging assailant's momentum.

Hand defenses are used when the assailant closes the distance quickly, takes the defender by surprise, or the defender is in a close-quarters situation. Note: Many students practice and emphasize hand defenses. However, when sparring against a facsimile edged-weapon attack, they quickly revert to and prefer leg defenses. Kick defenses also come naturally when facing an assailant threatening with the edged weapon but who remains uncommitted to the attack. Notably, spitting in the assailant's face as you launch your hand or leg defense is a tried, effective, proven tactic.

Regardless of the defense you use, even if you are slashed or stabbed, you must continue to fight. In training, you will probably be "nicked," slashed, or stabbed. Obviously, the goal is to improve your skill set to avoid being wounded at all let alone fatally slashed or stabbed. Again, if your defense is imperfect and you are stabbed or wounded, it is imperative that you press your defense and counterattack. Remember, you will fight as you train, so, try to train as you will fight. If you no longer resist, your attacker will likely continue to administer wounds that will, no doubt, be fatal. Puncture wounds initially feel like strikes and slashes might not be evident until you see your own blood.

Note that krav maga defenses against an edged weapon, broken bottle, or syringe are principally the same; however, the removal techniques from the assailant's grip may differ. Against a syringe, the defender must take extra care to avoid being stabbed because of blood borne pathogens or a drug's effects. Occasionally, the description edged weapon and knife are used interchangeably throughout the text to facilitate the flow of technique discussion. The next two chapters focus on edged-weapon defenses against the most common types of attacks; not every angle or direction is covered. Absorb the principles and apply them against variations not covered using good common sense along with a little trial and error if necessary.

Straight Kick Against an Overhead Attack

Author's Note: Due to photo constraints, in certain Chapter 3 techniques, the initial deflections-redirections are depicted, and while the final edged-weapon removal process is described, the photos are omitted. Be sure to understand thoroughly the Cavaliers #1 and #2 along with Control Holds A, B, and C (Chapter 1).

The most typical edged-weapon attack is an overhand lunging-type attack targeting the defender's neck area. The attack is best foiled at long range with a strong kick to the groin in combination with a body defense, especially when the assailant is charging at you.

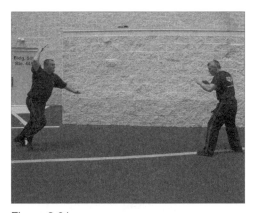

Figure 3.01a

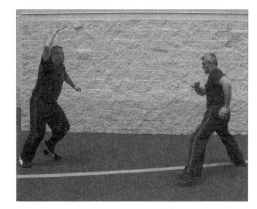

Figure 3.01b

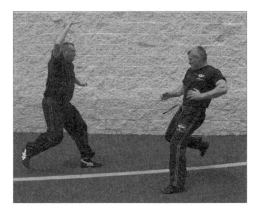

Figure 3.01c

Figures 3.01a–c. Most importantly, you must step off the line of attack to prevent the edged weapon from being plunged into you. With correct timing against a right-handed overhead attack, step off the line with your left leg turning out your left foot ninety degrees (opening up the base leg) allowing the right hip and your whole body maximum follow-through. Stepping out into the pivot also allows for glicha (Hebrew for a sliding step) to drive the kick through the opponent with your bodyweight generating optimum reach and power.

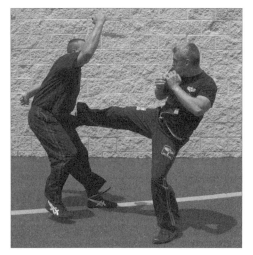

Figure 3.01d

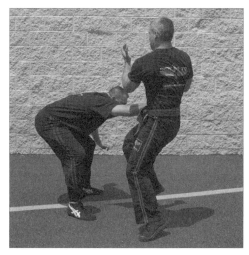

Figure 3.01e

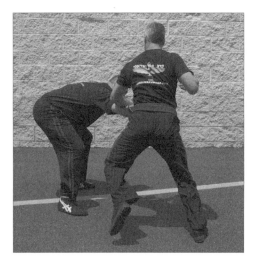

Figure 3.01f

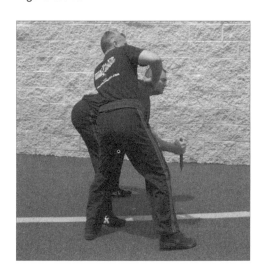

Figure 3.01g

Figures 3.01d–g. A full-force kick to the groin or midsection will jolt the attacker's body bringing his edged-weapon arm elbow back to his body. Keep in mind that a kick to the groin will generally lurch the upper body forward while stopping the body's progress at the hips. A kick to the torso will jolt the body backward. True to krav maga's philosophy of harnessing and honing the body's natural movements, the kicking leg will naturally retract on making contact. This is a crucial benefit because you retract the leg immediately to avoid being stabbed. This defense places you to the assailant's deadside to press the counterattack allowing another lowline sidekick to the assailant's knee, multiple punches to his head, and control of the edged-weapon arm with a wristlock or cavalier to remove the weapon or take the assailant down or both.

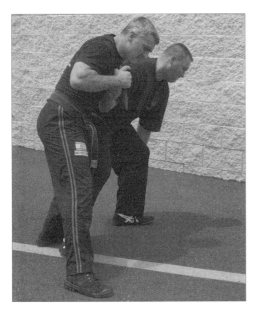

Figure 3.01h

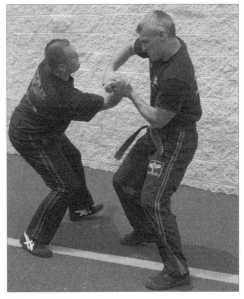

Figure 3.01i

Figures 3.01h–j. As learned previously in Figures 1.01a–y, use Cavalier #1 to take him down.

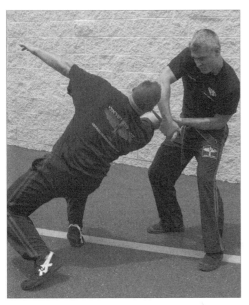

Figure 3.01j

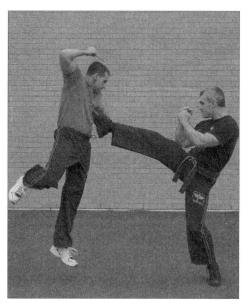

Figure 3.01k

Figure 3.01k. If the attacker jumps, use a straight defensive kick to his midsection or chest to drive him back. Follow-up with another immediate left kick to his groin. Subsequent defenses (covered just below) may be needed depending on the situation.

If the assailant has the edged weapon in his rear arm, another strong option to defend against the overhead attack is a sidekick to the assailant's lead knee with correct body lean and leg retraction followed by securing and taking away edged weapon with additional combatives similar to Figures 3.04a–c. Be sure to execute the sidekick by properly the turning base leg heel toward the assailant with proper body back lean with bodyweight forward to drive through the kick. These options take the defender's torso even farther away from the attack, but in the case of an overhead edged-weapon attack, retract the leg instantly to avoid the edged weapon potentially being plunged into your leg. Either continue the counterattack with additional kicks or close with hand defenses to secure the weapon. This lowline sidekick defense to the knee may be employed against any type of edged-weapon attack except an underhand stab (covered next).

A third less preferred option is to step off the line and "bail out" preferably to the assailant's deadside by delivering a debilitating roundhouse kick with the ball of the foot to the attacker's groin or shin to the assailant's midsection as depicted in Figure 3.03. Note: Again, if the leg is not withdrawn immediately, you are in jeopardy of the attacker's edged-weapon arm dropping quickly and impaling the leg. Again, you must press the counterattack with additional kicks or hand defenses, and close the distance to secure and remove the weapon.

Straight Kick Against an Underhand Attack

A second common edged attack is an underhand attack targeting your midsection or groin. The attack is best foiled at long range with a strong kick to either the head or the groin.

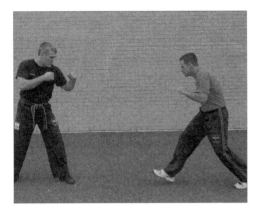

Figure 3.02a

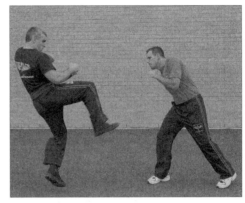

Figure 3.02b

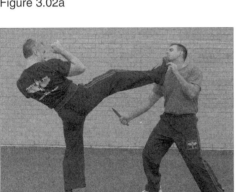

Figure 3.02c

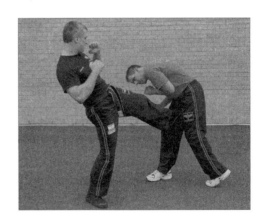

Figure 3.02d

Figures 3.02a–d. Optimally, you should kick the assailant in the face when he crouches to deliver the attack. However, not everyone can kick high to the head, so the defense may be modified with a kick to the groin. To take yourself off the line of attack and position yourself for the defensive kick, switch your feet by one foot replacing the other. Essentially, you are switching your feet. Against a right-handed underneath attack, your left foot will slide directly to the side to replace your right foot while the right hip chambers the right leg and swivels to deliver the straight kick. Keep your hands up in a protective position. Depending on your dexterity and timing, this can be considered a switch kick.

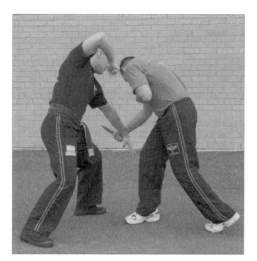

Figure 3.02e

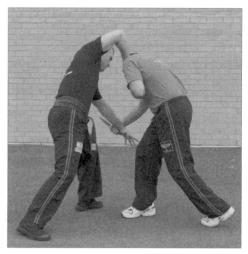

Figure 3.02f

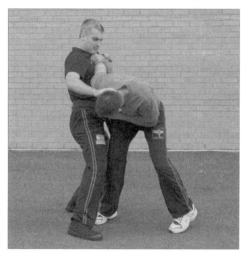

Figure 3.02g

Figures 3.02e–g. If your straight right kick knocks the assailant backward, immediately follow up with another swift left straight kick to the groin with proper base leg turn. If the initial kick does not reel him backward, immediately, follow-up with a left kick to his groin.

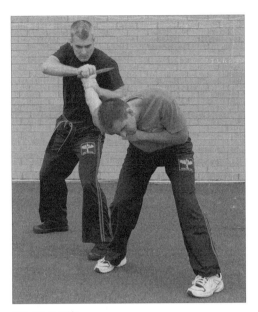

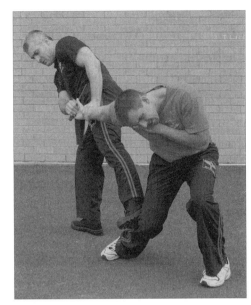

Figure 3.02h

Figure 3.02i

Figures 3.02h–i. After closing the distance to secure the weapon, deliver additional combatives and remove the weapon with one of your control hold options (Cavalier #2 depicted). Note: This defense may be used if an assailant is positioned in a left outlet stance and draws the edged weapon back to his hip in a threatening position but has not committed to an attack. You may wonder why you simply do not step off-line with your right foot and deliver a straight left kick. While this defense is possible, the leg switch generates more power and allows access to the attacker's head, depending on your flexibility. Lastly, you may not find yourself in a strong position to continue the counterattack to either engage or disengage.

Roundhouse Kick Against a Straight Stab

As with the previous two defenses, when defending against a straight stab, it is optimum to step off the line of attack while delivering a near-simultaneous counterattack. This defense uses a roundhouse kick with the ball of your foot to his groin or with the shin to the assailant's midsection. Notably, this kick can be used against straight punches, slashes, and hook stabs in keeping with krav maga's fundamental tenet, that of using one proven defense against myriad attacks. This defense operates on similar principles, the same as the previous leg defense against an overhead stab attack.

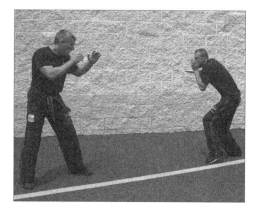

Figure 3.03a

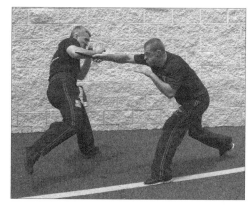

Figure 3.03b

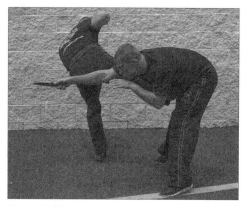

Figure 3.03c

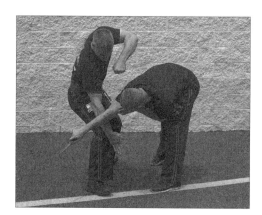

Figure 3.03d

Figures 3.03a–d. Step to the side with your outside arm held high to protect your head and deliver a roundhouse kick with the ball of the foot (curling your toes toward you) to the attacker's groin followed immediately by secure and take away the edged weapon with additional combatives as necessary. Keep your hands up in a protective position. Essentially, you are bailing out while keeping your hands up to deliver the lowline roundhouse-kick defense.

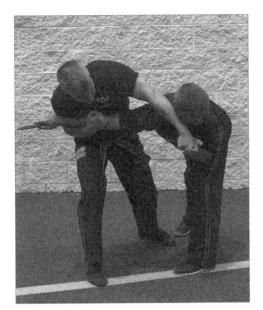

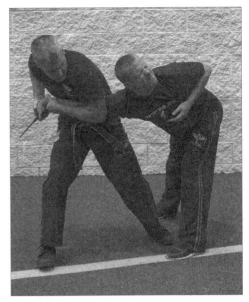

Figure 3.03e   Figure 3.03f

Figures 3.03e–f. Immediately follow up with additional kicks or close the distance to secure the edged weapon using a "police hold" or cavalier to take the assailant down. Alternatively, after the roundhouse kick, you may also use a lowline sidekick to the assailant's nearside knee. Note: This kick may also work against an overhead stab; however, immediately retract your leg to protect your leg from being impaled because this is a precision kick rather than a power kick.

Another option is a lowline sidekick to the attacker's knee. Drop your level below the attack and use your nearside hand to deflect as you destroy the assailant's knee.

Roundhouse Kick Against a Slash

Similar to defending a straight stab at the upper body in Figures 3.03a–f, defending against an inside or outside slash attack to your face or throat with your legs once again requires the defender to step off the line and deliver a roundhouse kick with the ball of the foot to the assailant's groin.

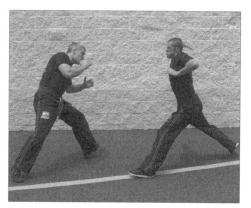

Figure 3.03g

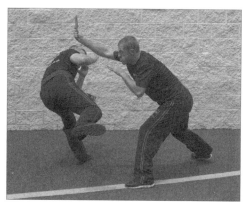

Figure 3.03h

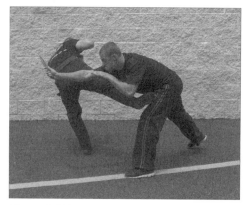

Figure 3.03i

Figures 3.03g–i. You must bail out while keeping your hands up to protect your throat and eyes against the slash and deliver the lowline roundhouse kick defense counterattack.

As in previous defenses, the main kick can be immediately followed up with an additional sidekick to the assailant's nearside knee. Follow up with a police hold or cavalier to take the assailant down. You may also use a low sidekick against assailant's knee, similar to kick defenses against regular or straight stab from side position.

Sidekick Against a High Straight Stab

A defensive option against a high straight stab attack is a lowline sidekick defense.

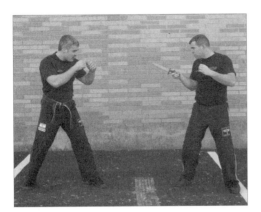

Figure 3.04a

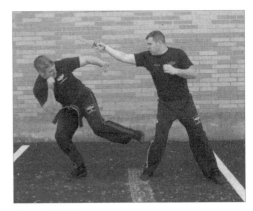

Figure 3.04b

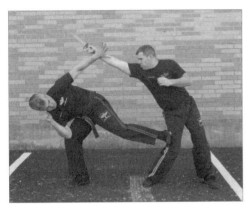

Figure 3.04c

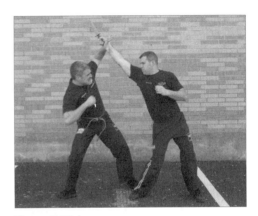

Figure 3.04d

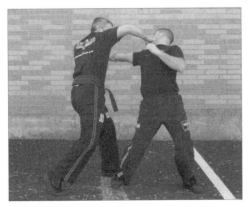

Figure 3.04e

Figures 3.04a–e. Execute the sidekick correctly leaning your body back and away from the incoming stab while turning your base leg heel transferring your weight to the ball of your foot. Strike with your heel preferably to his knee while using your forward hand in an upward motion as a secondary defense to ward off the stab. Finish with retzev combatives and Cavalier #2 or Police Hold A, or retreat. The sidekick defense can also be performed from the opposite stance.

Rear Stab Defenses

Attacking from the rear is a preferred method by assailants to surprise the defender with a stab in the back.

Overhead Attack

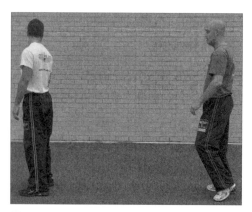 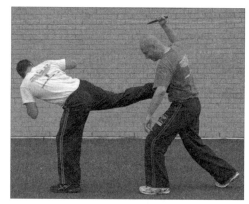

Figure 3.05a

Figure 3.05b

Figures 3.05a–b. This defense uses a strong debilitating rear defensive kick with the heel against the assailant's groin or midsection to stop the attack. The defender must immediately withdraw the leg and turn to press the attack with additional kicks or hand defenses to close the distance combined with additional combatives to secure the weapon. Another smart option—as with all edged-weapon defenses—is to simply run. An additional tactic requiring mention if you are stabbed, krav maga uses a combat roll forward to then turn and face the attacker to defend or to keep running. The goal is never to get stabbed, but if you are stabbed once, not to absorb multiple wounds.

Defending a Surprise Short Straight Stab

This defense is an instinctive late defense when the assailant has managed to come very close to you and attempts a short straight stab into your midsection.

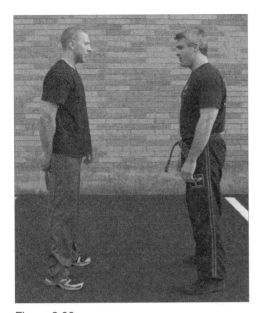

Figure 3.06a

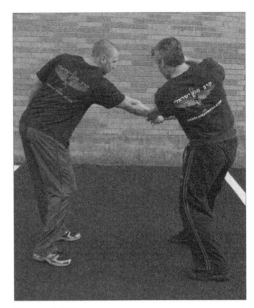

Figure 3.06b

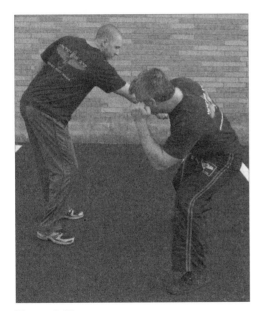

Figure 3.06c

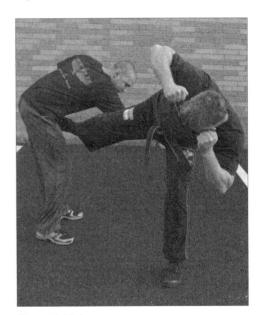

Figure 3.06d

Figures 3.06a–d. Use a deflection-redirection and simultaneous body defense combined with a roundhouse kick using the ball of your foot (curling your toes toward you) directed into the assailant's groin, or shin kick to the midsection. With your sameside hand as the assailant's weapon arm, parry the edged weapon away with your palm keeping all of your fingers together while stepping to the outside opposite of your parry to deliver the kick.

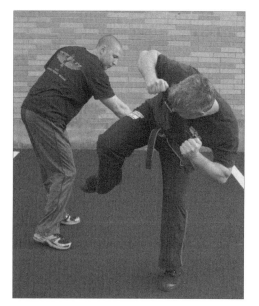

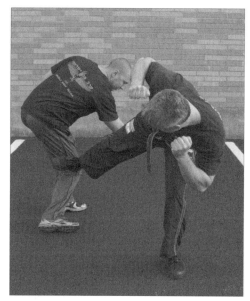

Figure 3.06e

Figure 3.06f

Figures 3.06e–f. You can also add a rapid-fire sidekick with your same kicking leg to the assailant's nearside knee to either escape or close the distance to secure the edged weapon arm while continuing your retzev counterattack and disarm. Close on the attacker with a block and trap, administering a simultaneous counterattack to the head. Cavalier #1 or Control Hold C are good options to take the assailant down.

Note: The upper body element of this defense is used if you were on the ground, struggling from your back against an assailant with your shin/knee brace keeping distance, and he suddenly deploys an edged weapon and attempts a short stab to your groin or midsection. Because of the body positioning and the attacker's proximity to you, this is a difficult defense requiring immediate recognition and action.

Using Shield-like Objects Against an Edged-Weapon Attack

Use a bag, briefcase, book, magazine, or any other object to parry or block the attack while delivering a simultaneous kick followed by retzev counterattacks.

The best strategy is to use a combined deflection-redirection and body defense with a simultaneous roundhouse kick to the assailant's groin or knee.

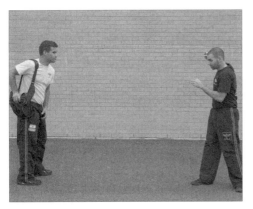

Figure 3.07a

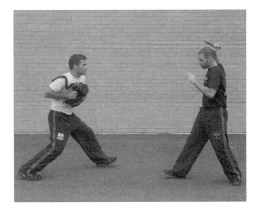

Figure 3.07b

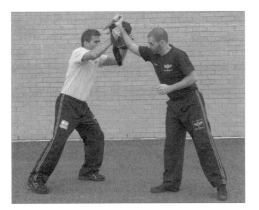

Figure 3.07c

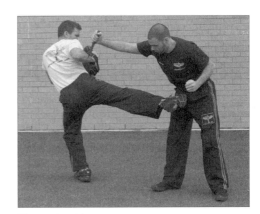

Figure 3.07d

Figures 3.07a–d. Try to step off the line of attack away from the threat using the shield at an angle to deflect/redirect the attack rather than using force against force to block it. Angling your deflection-redirection to send the attack off to the side takes you to the assailant's deadside providing a better tactical position. A glicha (sliding step) will also help generate more movement behind the kick. You could follow up with a sidekick to the assailant's nearside knee, use the shield to batter him, or launch the shield at him and close on him to control the weapon and remove it.

Defending an Attacker Using Two Edged Weapons

Defending against an attacker who is using two of his edged weapons interchangeably or alternating his stabs and slashes is difficult. Leg defenses combined with some kind or shield or barrier to block the attack while kicking underneath are the best answer. However, the attacker can stab or slash at your legs, especially if he is using a reverse grip on one or both of the weapons. You must always attempt to move to the attacker's deadside. Again, note that moving to the deadside of a skilled opponent can be extremely difficult as he can simply pivot away from you and continue his attack.

Edged-Weapon Threats

Defending Against an Assailant Posturing/Threatening with an Edged Weapon

An assailant may threaten you with an edged weapon from different ranges. Here we examine "leg range" threats.

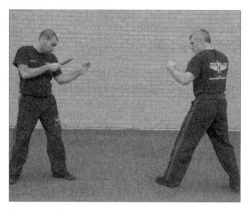

Figure 3.08a

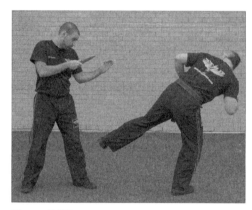

Figure 3.08b

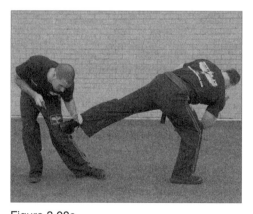

Figure 3.08c

Figures 3.08a–c. A lowline sidekick or straight kick targeting the assailant's knees or groin can be highly effective when combined with a distraction. Be aware, however, that a skilled edged-weapon fighter can simply and quickly slash or stab down at your incoming leg, especially, if he has an "icepick" grip that allows him to lower the weapon quickly. After disabling his knee, retreat.

Defending When the Assailant Switches the Edged Weapon Between His Hands

This defense requires timing to deliver a straight kick to the assailant's groin as he switches control of the edged weapon from hand to hand.

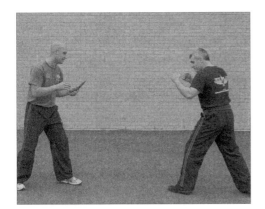

Figure 3.09a

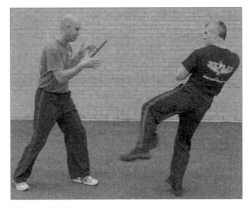

Figure 3.09b

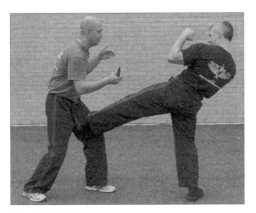

Figure 3.09c

Figures 3.09a–c. With correct timing, a debilitating straight kick with the ball of the foot to the assailant's groin or knee is a strong defense. A sidekick may also be used. Either escape or close to control the assailant. Keep in mind the edged weapon may fall to ground, but the priority is to control or debilitate the assailant. Of course, be aware of any third party who may retrieve the weapon to use against you. We hope that your awareness training will alert you to this, but you may also use the assailant as a shield with the correct control holds. Continue to press your attacks as necessary. Either close on the attacker to control and remove the weapon, or retreat.

An Assailant Posturing with an Edged Weapon at a Distance

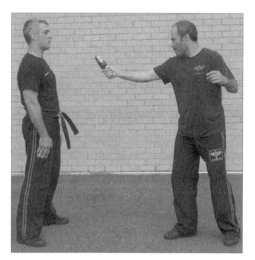

Figure 3.10a

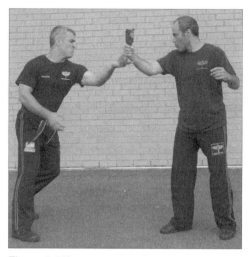

Figure 3.10b

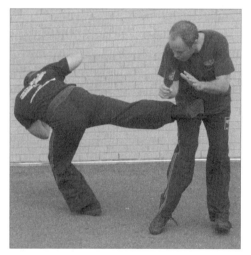

Figure 3.10c

Figures 3.10a–c. An assailant might posture with a edged weapon such as in a mugging situation. He might also pull out an edged weapon for intimidation while remaining momentarily ambivalent if he truly wants to escalate the situation. You cannot be ambivalent. Any person holding an edged weapon in front of you represents a life-threatening situation. De-escalation by talking him down may work, but if you judge the person intends you imminent bodily harm, react decisively. If possible, forcefully slap the assailant's weapon hand or wrist to redirect the weapon away from you. Debilitate the assailant with a lowline kick.

Alternatively, overcome the threat using whatever technique or weapon of opportunity is at your disposal. Generally, a distraction, if handy, such as throwing loose change or spitting in the assailant's face combined with an immediate straight, side, or roundhouse kick is highly effective. Either immediately close the distance to him with simultaneous additional combatives and control of the weapon arm, or retreat.

When using a distraction, your object(s) should be hidden in the hand or not otherwise displayed to preserve your advantage and should be timed to launch with the simultaneous kick. Finish the defense and control the weapon moving to the deadside. While not recommended, advanced students may combine a distraction with a strong slap kick with the instep of the foot to the back of the assailant's hand to dislodge the edged weapon. To be sure, this is a particularly risky tactic if the assailant has quick reflexes or you telegraph your intention and movement.

Defenses When the Defender Is on the Ground

You could find yourself initially in an unarmed ground fight and have it rapidly escalate into an edged-weapon attack. In other words, if you are winning an unarmed battle, your adversary might try to compensate by deploying a previously hidden weapon.

As in a standing fight, there is a strong possibility that you may not realize the fight has instantaneously changed from an unarmed confrontation into an armed attack. There are several places an assailant might hide a weapon including the small of his back, his waistband, his boot or sock, or his sleeve among other places.

Krav maga's defensive principles remain the same when defending an upright attack or a ground attack. Deflect-redirect, use a body defense when possible, and counterattack simultaneously and relentlessly. When facing a weapon, attacking your opponent's vital anatomy is paramount. Striking the assailant in the eyes, throat, and groin may preempt his ability to deploy a weapon, especially, when he is reaching for it. However, use of your legs and body defenses naturally change when on the ground. In addition, you could find yourself on the ground fighting against a standing assailant who is slashing and stabbing at your legs. He might also be looking for the opportunity to fall and impale you with his edged weapon, using all of his bodyweight. The key again, as with krav maga's standing defenses, is when possible move your body off the line of attack.

Both the Assailant and Defender Are on the Ground

If the assailant does deploy the edged weapon, your legs can be highly effective defensive weapons to create separation in combination with powerful leg combatives. In addition, if you are able to place your foot on his edged-weapon wielding shoulder, you can effectively control his movements while counterattacking his head, eyes, throat, solar plexus, and groin with your other leg to create separation and escape.

Defending Against a Standing Assailant Slashing at Your Legs or Jumping on You

If the assailant is standing and you are on your back, lowline straight kicks may be used to hobble the assailant's knees. Optimally, you will attack his knee on the opposite side of his edged-weapon hand. You can also attack his groin with a straight kick. It is also possible to disable the assailant with a sharp sidekick to his nearest ankle. As always, your defensive timing must be correct. Be aware if your preemptive or defensive kicks are not properly timed, you are vulnerable to severe leg wounds. If the assailant is looking for an opening to launch himself onto you with the edged weapon, use good body transition and legwork with strong kicks to his groin or midsection retracting them quickly. Follow up with additional kicks to his vulnerable areas to keep him from landing on you. If you succeed with an initial strong kick and can get up to escape, do it.

Overhead Attack Defense When the Defender is on His Back

An assailant may deploy an edged weapon in a ground fight. If the assailant is on top of the defender, gravity enhances the force of the downward attack. Unlike a standing position, a body defense is not as effective because of the nature of groundfighting; the defender's mobility is more restricted.

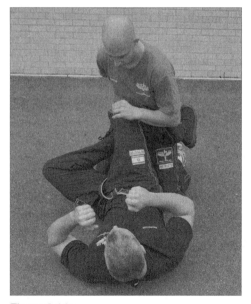
Figure 3.11a

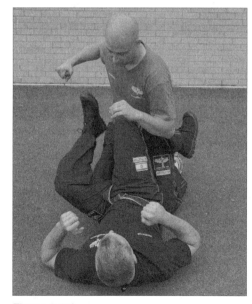
Figure 3.11b

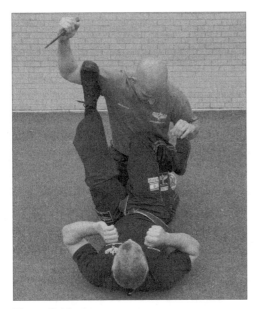
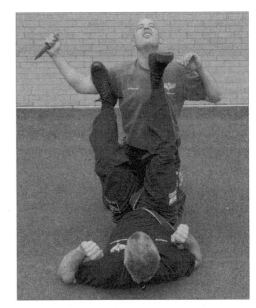

Figure 3.11c   Figure 3.11d

Figures 3.11a–d. When the defender is on his back and the assailant is on his knees, the preferred krav maga position (in any groundfight when the defender has his back to the ground) is to use a diagonal knee brace across the assailant's chest with your opposite foot on the assailant's sameside hip. If you are on your back and the assailant deploys an edged weapon, a highly effective defense is to place your nearside foot on his edged-weapon wielding shoulder. Your legs house your most powerful muscle groups. Jolting your assailant backward helps you create separation and the opportunity to kick him in the head, solar plexus, or groin multiple times. Keep your hands up in case he is able to overcome your initial leg defense. Note: While the high closed guard (when the defender wraps his legs around the assailant's waist) will hinder the assailant's mobility, it is not failsafe against an assailant reaching and successfully deploying a concealed weapon. In addition, if the assailant maintains his posture he can pummel and then stab you in the groin.

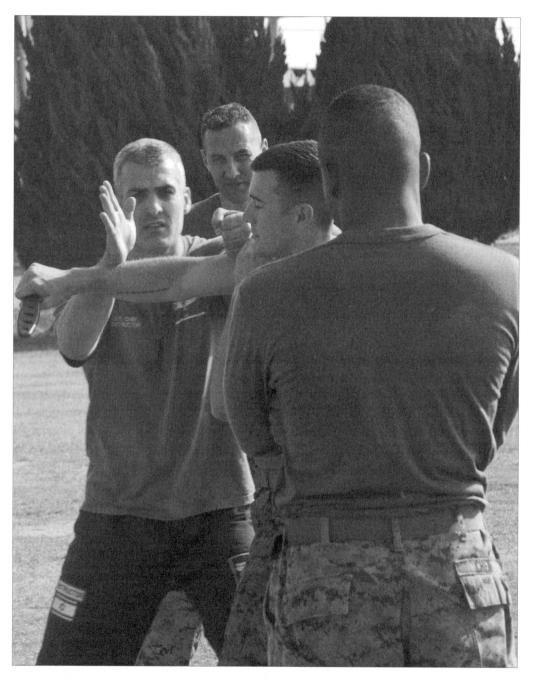

Training U.S. Marines. Photo courtesy of USMC Combat Camera.

CHAPTER 4

Hand Defenses Against Edged Weapons

Hand defenses are used when (1) the assailant closes the distance; (2) you are in a close-quarters combat situation; or (3) you are surprised by the attack.

Author's Note: Due to space constraints, for some Chapter 4 techniques, the initial deflections-redirections are depicted, and while explained, the final edged-weapon removal photos are omitted. Be sure to understand thoroughly the Cavaliers #1 and #2 along with Control Holds A, B, and C (Chapter 1.)

Defending an Incoming Overhead Stab

This defense thwarts the most typical edged-weapon attack, the overhead stab, when you are too close for leg defenses. In other words, you do not recognize the attack early enough to use leg defenses or find yourself in a confined space where leg defenses are not an option.

As noted, all krav maga weapon defenses, when possible, move off the line of attack combined with defense and attack. This defense primarily relies on your instinct to block and move away from a blow, or, in this case, a stab. The defender does not have time to stop the attacker's arm as he draws it back to stab.

The assailant has the edged weapon in his right hand and is facing you. This attack can involve tremendous force as the assailant presses all of his weight into the attack and uses gravity to his advantage. The defense involves a simultaneous three-part movement.

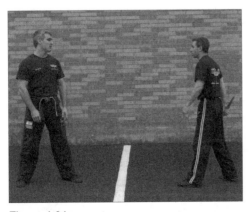

Figure 4.01a

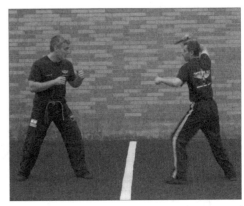

Figure 4.01b

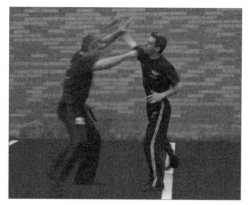

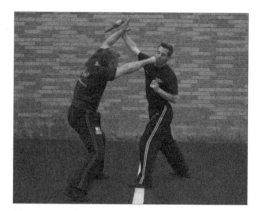

Figure 4.01c   Figure 4.01d

Figures 4.01a–d. You must (1) deflect-redirect the assailant's right-edged weapon hand using an outside block by rotating your left arm (nearest to the edged weapon) outside to intercept the assailant's right arm while not breaking contact for control; (2) simultaneously strike the assailant in the face or throat with your right hand, as you (3) step forward and diagonally with your outside right leg taking you off the line of attack and into weapon control.

Recall that krav maga's defenses must work for everyone and do not rely on strength. When confronting a larger stronger assailant, if you do not step out off the line of attack, this disparity in body mass and strength could overcome your arm block even if you throw your bodyweight behind it. If you simply "burst" into the attacker, there is a considerable risk you will be stabbed (or in a different attack, slashed). Stepping out takes you off the line of attack and will work against an overhead long edged weapon or a machete stab. When using a strong block, you may find that your hand naturally curves slightly upward.

Strive to deflect the edged weapon as close as possible to the assailant's wrist while maintaining contact with the assailant's arm after the initial block. After stunning the assailant, you have the option of pressing the counterattack by transitioning immediately from the block to securing the assailant's arm. In other words, block the attack by rotating your left arm outward and then immediately slightly rotate the arm back to grab and secure the assailant's right wrist. This is done while stepping slightly to the side and away from the assailant. Immediately secure the assailant's arm and drive it back while delivering punishing knee strikes to the groin or thighs. Keep in mind, after the deflection and without attempting to control the arm, you may simply kick him in the groin and retreat.

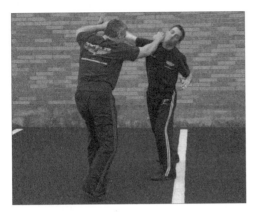

Figure 4.01e

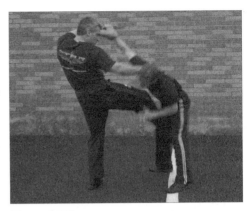

Figure 4.01f

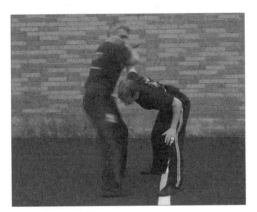

Figure 4.01g

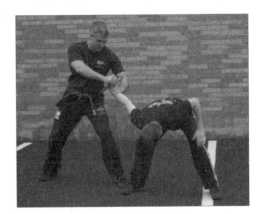

Figure 4.01h

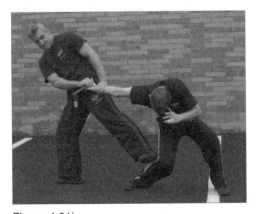

Figure 4.01i

Figures 4.01e–i. It is paramount that after you take a step away from the attack **to then drive** the assailant's arm backward for control. After stepping off the line of attack, driving the assailant's arm back serves two purposes: (1) it prevents the assailant from initiating further stabs, and (2) it positions the defender to apply a strong control hold, in this case the options of Control Holds A or Cavalier #1. Control Hold A (known to some as the "kimura") secures the assailant, driving him face-down, importantly placing strong control over the edged-weapon hand. Control the edged weapon and remove it with precision from the assailant's grip. Secure the weapon at the bottom of the hilt and

Figures 4.01j–p. Caption continue on next page

pry it loose with your right thumb from the assailant's grip toward his head. Another option is to keep the assailant's elbow pinned to your body and release your left hand from the attacker's wrist and inserting your thumb to pry the edged weapon.

You should remember that kravists train to use wrist releases and scissor leg takedowns. In a fight, An assailant could use the same release against you. Wrist releases, when holding a blade, present special dangers because not only can the assailant release, he can slash and stab while doing it.

You may also use Cavalier #2 to remove the edged weapon and remain standing (depicted in Figures 4.06i–p).

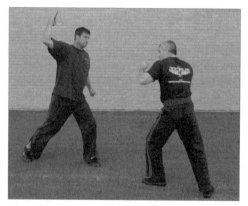

Figure 4.01j

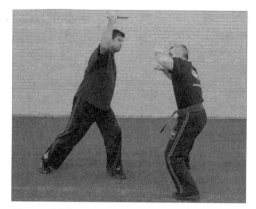

Figure 4.01k

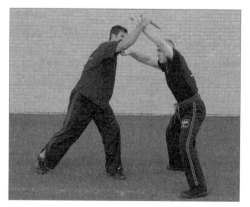

Figure 4.01l

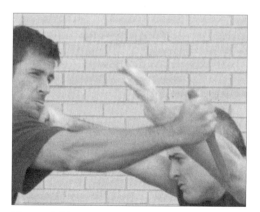

Figure 4.01m

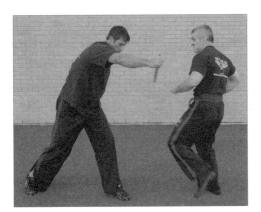

Figure 4.01n

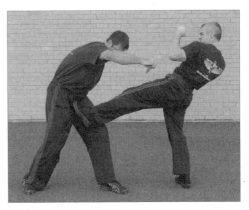

Figure 4.01o

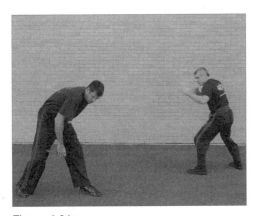

Figure 4.01p

Figures 4.01j–p. A second option to defend the attack uses the primary defense to block/sidestep and counterattack but breaks contact to deliver a swift, strong, left straight kick to the groin with a good base leg turn. This is a strong option because the attacker's arm will bounce off your deflecting arm and can be difficult to control. The sidestep places your right leg forward with your weight on it to take you off the line of attack. Because the step shifts your weight to your right leg, your left leg is positioned to deliver a debilitating left straight kick to the assailant's groin. This shift, in turn, allows you to quickly disengage while continuing to break the angle (moving away from the edged weapon). For law enforcement, security, and professional security personnel, this variation also allows you to deploy a firearm or impact weapon you did not originally have time to use.

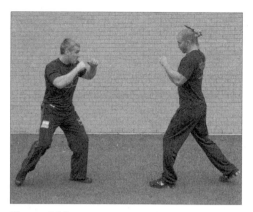

Figure 4.01q

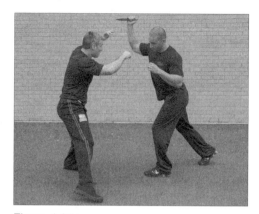

Figure 4.01r

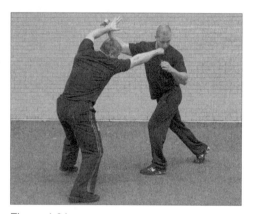

Figure 4.01s

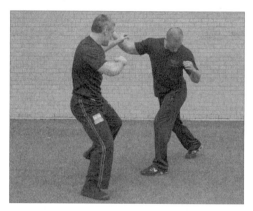

Figure 4.01t

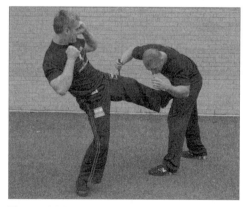

Figure 4.01u

Figures 4.01q–u. The defense shown from the opposite view.

A third law enforcement, professional security, or military specific option is to complete the block/sidestep and counterattack, and then immediately draw and instinctively point shoot the assailant. Note: Blocking and simultaneously drawing the weapon is not an optimum tactic because the assailant is coming at you full speed and force, likely with repeated stabs, and you have not yet stunned him. Instead, you are relying on your ability to deploy and successfully use your weapon, which, unfortunately, has had fatal consequences for many police and security officers. (A different technique must be used if the defender has the sidearm on his left hip.) You should continue to move away from the edged-weapon arm. In short, this defense can be combined with an initial strike to momentarily stun the assailant, create distance, and then deploy a firearm.

A fourth option developed by Grandmaster Gidon is to step off the line of attack and deliver an over-top-knuckles punch to the eye ridge or palm-heel strike to the ear while the continuing tsai-bake movement away from the attack to retreat and escape.

Overhead Defense When Not "Nose to Nose" or the Defender Can Burst Early

If an assailant is facing you positioned slightly to your left (not directly in front of you as depicted in Figures 4.01a–g) and he attempts an overhead stab, you will likely not have time to step off the line of attack (the previous defense) because of the short distance to the edged-weapon arm.

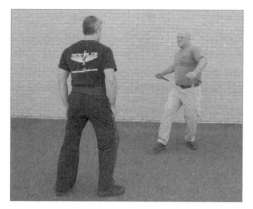

Figure 4.02a

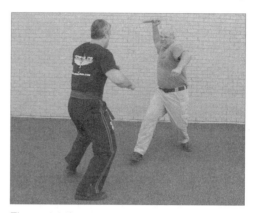

Figure 4.02b

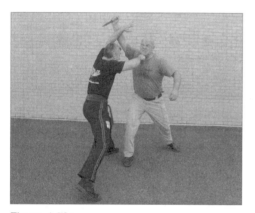

Figure 4.02c

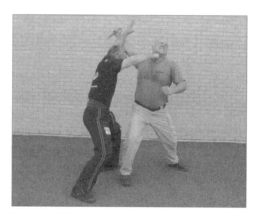

Figure 4.02d

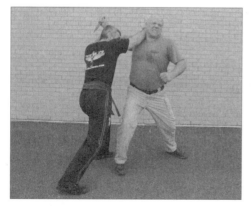

Figure 4.02e

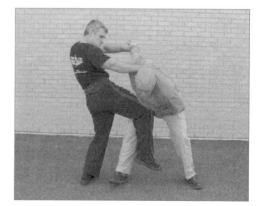

Figure 4.02f

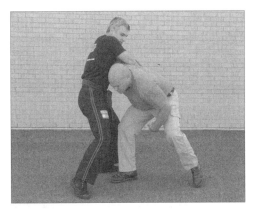

Figure 4.02g

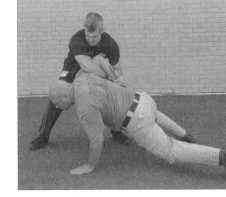

Figure 4.02h

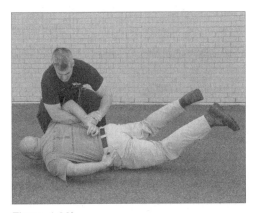

Figure 4.02i

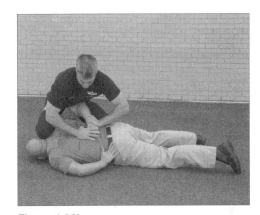

Figure 4.02j

Figures 4.02a–j. In this defense, you are in a position to block and attack by bursting into the assailant directly transferring your entire bodyweight against the incoming edged weapon arm while counterstriking. You have the advantage of propelling your bodyweight behind the block to drive the edged-weapon arm shoulder back to secure the weapon while delivering additional combatives including devastating knee strikes. In addition, this defense can be used if you are "nose to nose" with the assailant and you recognize the attack early enough to close the distance. In other words, you can catch the attacker as he draws the edged weapon back and coils his shoulder. Close the distance and continue to administer combatives until the attacker is no longer a threat. Use Control Hold A or Cavalier #2 to remove the weapon. Notably, some people may wish to attempt Cavalier #1. However, you must change grips and then bring the blade across your body, which is not a preferred option.

As previously noted, a common serious mistake is to use the direct bursting technique into the assailant's weapon arm shoulder when aligned face to face with the assailant, and his attacking arm has forward momentum. A small defender will not be able to defend against a large powerful assailant because of the disparity in strength and body mass coupled with the gravity of the downward strike arcing toward the defender. Remember, krav maga defenses must work for everyone.

Defending an Overhead Off-Angle Stab When Facing in Opposite Direction

An assailant might be to side of you and launch and overhead attack.

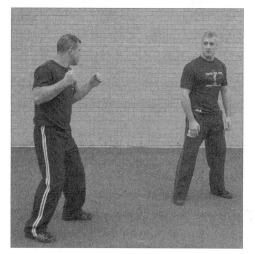

Figure 4.03a

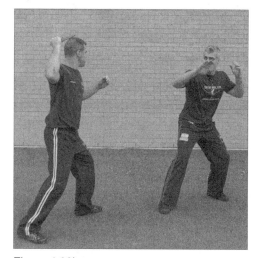

Figure 4.03b

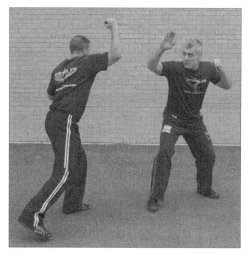

Figure 4.03c

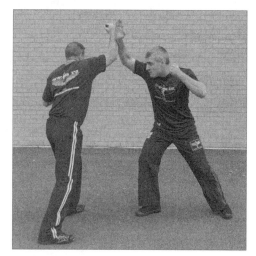

Figure 4.03d

Figures 4.03a–d. Again, this defense relies on our instinct to block and move away from a blow or stab. The defense involves an outside rotational block with the forearm (ulna) while stepping off-line toward the assailant with your farside leg pivoting one-hundred-eighty degrees. You should try to deflect the edged weapon as close as possible to the assailant's wrist.

Following the initial deflect-redirect switch arms immediately to control the weapon. This "closing technique" brings you to the assailant's deadside, allowing for multiple body punches to the assailant's head. Do not break contact with the attacker's arm to maintain control. Secure the assailant's wrist with his elbow pinned against your torso making sure to stay well inside the edged weapon's arc by keeping your torso nearly parallel with his torso. After the assailant ceases to be a threat, you may transition to Cavalier #1 to remove the weapon or the Face and Weapon control hold.

Straight Stab "L" Block

This defense allows you to deflect an incoming left- or right-handed straight stab from either outlet stance while simultaneously stepping off the line of attack, trapping your opponent's arm, and delivering your own straight punch counterattacks to the attacker's throat, chin, or nose.

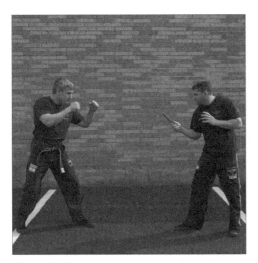

Figure 4.04a

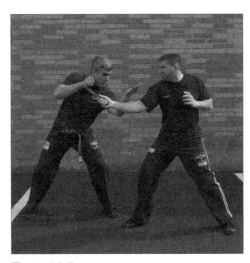

Figure 4.04b

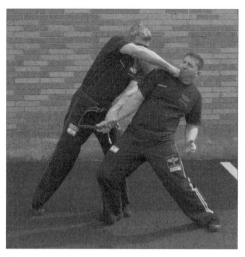

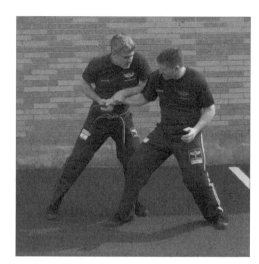

Figure 4.04c

Figure 4.04d

Figures 4.04a–d. From your regular left outlet stance, your left arm leads the body to parry the thrust as you sidestep. The arm should be bent at an approximately seventy- degree angle to deflect-redirect the assailant's straight stab while making a subtle sidestep to the left. The parrying movement is no more than four- to six-inches because it leads the body's defensive movement—as with most krav maga defensive tactics. This deflection-redirection is not an uncontrolled swipe or grab at the assailant's incoming arm (a common mistake when first learning the technique). The defensive arm makes uses of the entire length of the forearm or from the pinky to the elbow to deflect any change in the height of the opponent's stab attempt. The movement rotates the wrist outward so that your left thumb, kept attached to the hand with all the fingers pointing up, turns away from you as contact is made with the opponent's arm to redirect the incoming thrust. Do not break contact with the edged-weapon arm even if you cannot secure the arm, pin it to the attacker's torso and continue your retzev counterattacks. Keep in mind the assailant may lunge bringing you deep into his deadside as he closes the distance while you simultaneously step off line. After the parry is made and without breaking contact with the assailant's arm, which he will most likely retract, hook the assailant's arm by cupping your left hand, wrapping your left thumb around his forearm for control, and pinning the arm against the assailant's torso while delivering debilitating counterpunches to the throat or jaw. Note again, the assailant may generate such momentum that you deflect and move deep into his deadside. Nevertheless, do not break contact with the edged-weapon arm even if you cannot secure the arm and continue your retzev counterattacks. You are still safe provided you are inside the attack arc (usually a backstab or backslash) of the edged weapon. While pressing your counterattack, you can secure the edged-weapon arm with your right arm and take the assailant down using a fishhook into his eye, neck crank, or other combative.

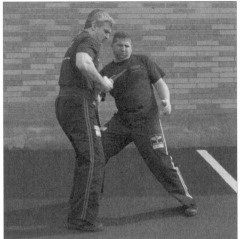

Figure 4.04e

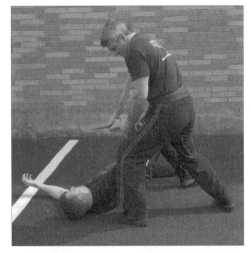

Figure 4.04f

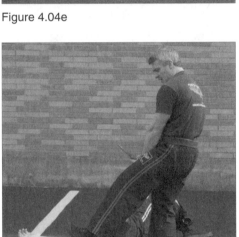

Figure 4.04g

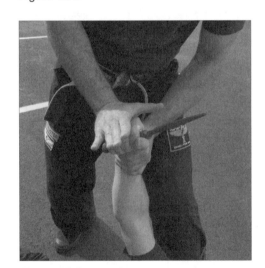

Figure 4.04h

Figures 4.04e–h. The objective is avoid being stabbed while placing you to the assailant's deadside with simultaneous combatives setting up Cavalier #1 into additional retzev counterattacks, including a powerful takedown, stomps to the head, and pealing the edged weapon from the assailant's grip or turning the assailant over to restrain him and removing the weapon.

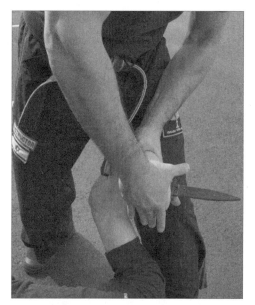

Figure 4.04i

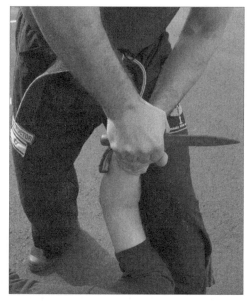

Figure 4.04j

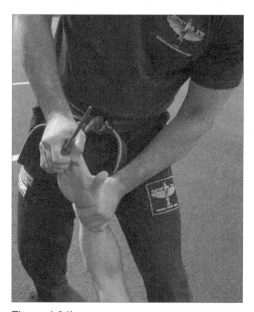

Figure 4.04k

Figures 4.04i–k. To remove the weapon from his grip, use the palm heel of your "knuckles to knuckles" hand to punch his wrist toward him using your hips and upper body in concert. For added power, you may momentarily release your grip to cock your arm slightly to palm heel through his wrist. You can also deliver an elbow strike to his wrist, but use careful aim not to lacerate yourself on the edged weapon. As you break the wrist's posture, dig your fingers into his palm wrapping around the weapon's grip. Use your fingers to strip the weapon and pry it from his grip.

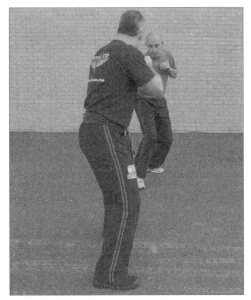

Figure 4.04l

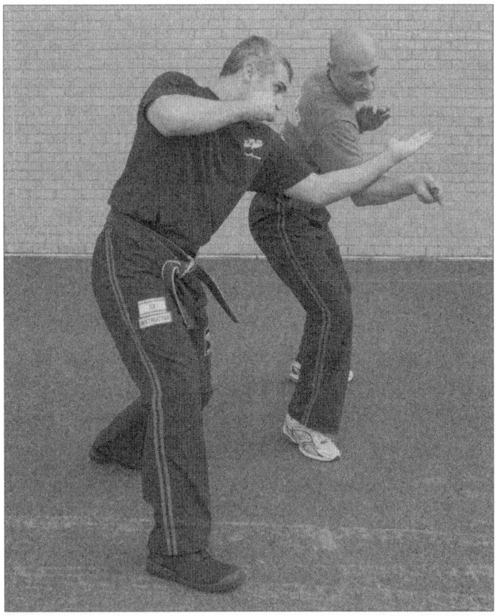

Figure 4.04m

Figures 4.04l–m. Rear view of the initial defense.

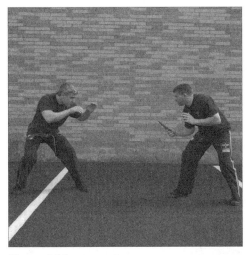

Figure 4.04n

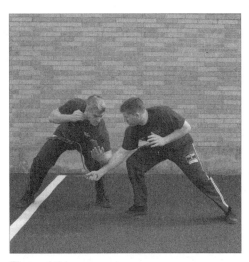

Figure 4.04o

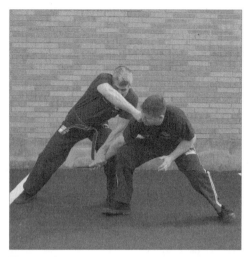

Figure 4.04p

Figures 4.04n–p. The technique is the same for defending against a low stab; however, you must drop your level by bending your knees to the opponent's level. Beware of feints where the opponent initially motions low and then stabs high. Feints with a knife are very difficult to defend. You must be prepared with the correct body positioning and an understanding of the most natural feints—armed or unarmed for that matter.

Bonus: this defense can also used to defend against a straight punch.

Straight Stab "L" Block When in an Opposite Outlet Stance

This defense, similar to the previous technique, allows you deflect an incoming straight stab and step off the line of attack when you find yourself in a right outlet stance and your opponent is in a left outlet stance.

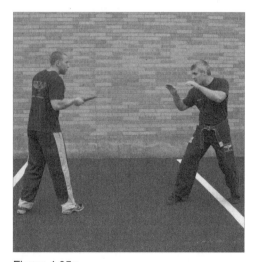

Figure 4.05a

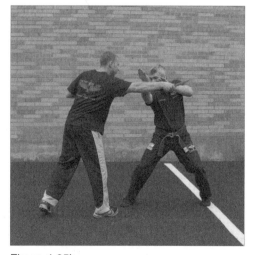

Figure 4.05b

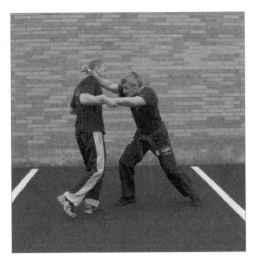

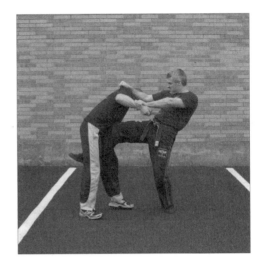

Figure 4.05c

Figure 4.05d

Figures 4.05a–d. From your regular right outlet stance, your right arm leads the body to parry. The arm should be bent at an approximately seventy degree angle to deflect-redirect the assailant's straight stab while making a subtle sidestep to the right taking you off the line of attack. The parrying movement leads the body's defensive movement that naturally moves the torso off the line of attack. The deflection-redirection is no more than a four- to six-inch movement diagonally out; the defensive movement is not an uncontrolled swipe. After the parry is made, rotate the right arm back and deliver an outside chop (or hammerfist) to the assailant's neck while securing the opponent's weapon arm with your left hand. Your parry will force his weapon arm outward and he will begin to retract it, so you must secure his arm instantaneously using the correct timing. Continue with retzev, delivering a right knee to groin, a right horizontal elbow to the throat, or a vertical elbow to the back of the neck followed by additional retzev combatives or a Police Control Hold A.

To control the edged weapon with precision, it is also possible to defend using a simultaneous outside chop and sameside knee strike to the groin. Note: This defense builds the foundation for krav maga's defenses against several edged-weapons attacks using an impact weapon wielded by the defender's forward arm.

Instinctive Defense Against a Close Underhand Stab

This defense is used when the defender does not recognize the attack until the last possible moment, hence, its instinctive name.

Optimally, awareness training would not allow anyone to come within attack range, especially if his or her hands are concealed.

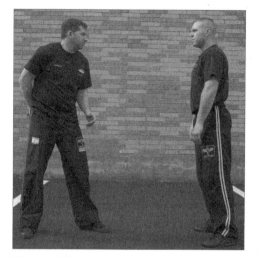

Figure 4.06a

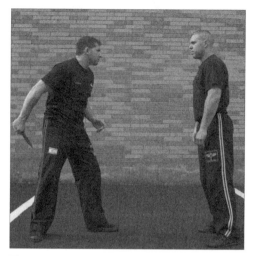

Figure 4.06b

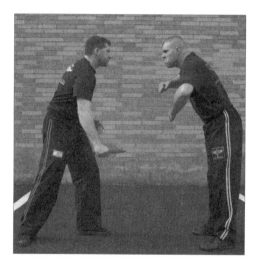

Figure 4.06c

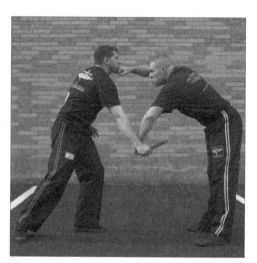

Figure 4.06d

Figures 4.06a–d. Use a simultaneous block and counterattack to the face, jaw, or throat while not breaking contact from the weapon arm. The block requires a ninety-degree bend of your elbow and a hollowing out of the hips while you deliver a counterstrike and move to control the weapon. A common mistake is to have one leg lowered and the other leg back. The counterstrike should stun your assailant and allow you to press the counterattack. The blocking arm should target just above the assailant's wrist or where one would normally wear a wristwatch.

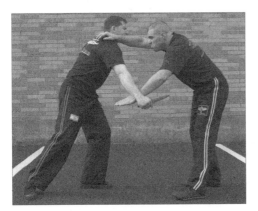

Figure 4.06e

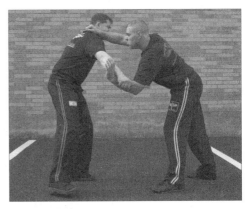

Figure 4.06f

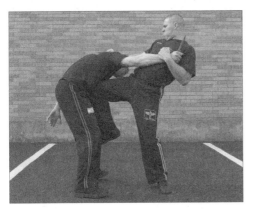

Figure 4.06g

Figures 4.06e–g. After the block and punch are delivered, the blocking arm, without breaking contact with the assailant's arm, snakes up and around the assailant's arm pulling it securely into your chest for maximum control of the weapon. Be sure to keep the edged weapon away from your throat and head as you execute this snaking motion while delivering multiple debilitating knee strikes to the assailant's groin.

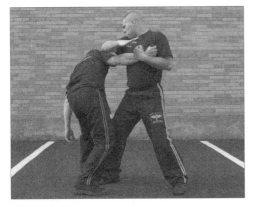

Figure 4.06h

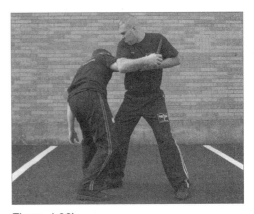

Figure 4.06i

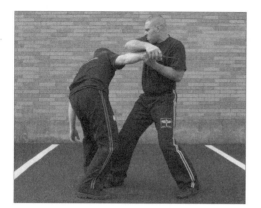

Figure 4.06j

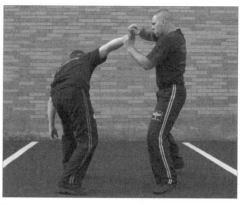

Figure 4.06k

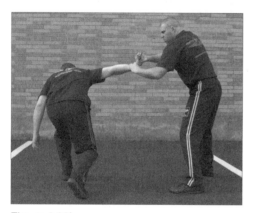

Figure 4.06l

Figures 4.06h–l. To remove the weapon, you may use a number of options including Control Hold A or Cavalier #2. Once you have stopped the attack and sufficiently debilitated the assailant with combatives to establish firm control over his weapon arm, reach your hand across your chest to grab the back of the assailant's hand placing the flat of your hand over the back of his hand. This creates a "knuckles to knuckles" position. By positioning your knuckles down ("thumb to you") with your palm against the back flat side of his hand ("prayer" hold) with your opposite hand also facing down and parallel, rotate the assailant's hand down and away by taking a tsai-bake step. You know where the assailant's hand is positioned so you need not look at it. Keep your eyes on the assailant allowing you to pan for additional threats. A devastating finish to this technique is a sidekick to the assailant's nearside knee. Be sure to keep your elbows tight to your torso to maintain maximum control over the attacker's weapon arm and, when turning, keep the blade away from you. In other words, do not bring the blade across your throat or face while rotating his arm.

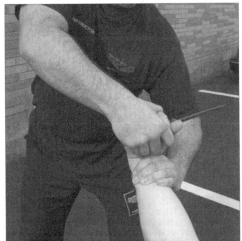

Figure 4.06m

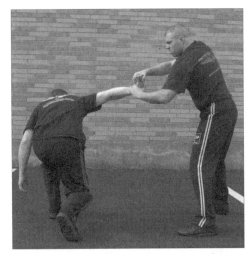

Figure 4.06n

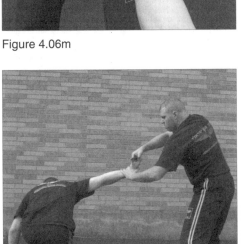

Figure 4.06o

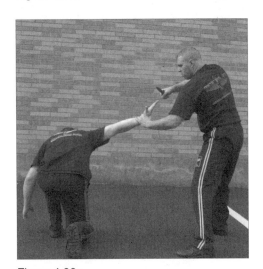

Figure 4.06p

Figures 4.06m–p. To remove the weapon from his grip, use the palm heel of your "knuckles to knuckles" hand to punch his wrist toward him using your hips and upper body in concert. For added power, you may momentarily release your grip to cock your arm slightly to palm heel through his wrist. As you break the wrist's posture, dig your fingers into his palm wrapping around the weapon's grip. Use your fingers to strip the weapon and pry it from his grip.

A third variation, Cavalier #3, involves maintaining strong control of the arm and rotating the attacker's arm with your right arm to force the tip of the weapon down allowing you to peel the weapon away.

Sidestep an Underhand Stab

This defense is used when the defender recognizes an incoming underhand attack.

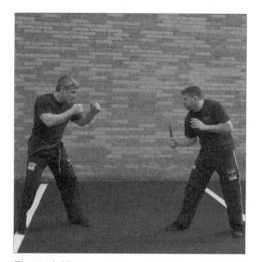

Figure 4.07a

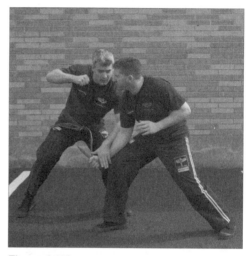

Figure 4.07b

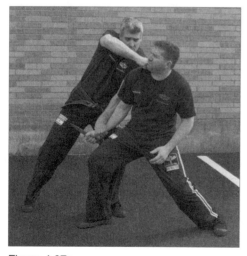

Figure 4.07c

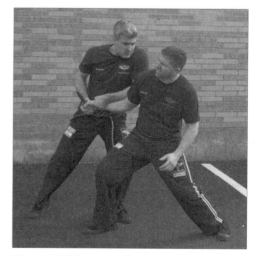

Figure 4.07d

Figures 4.07a–e. Caption on next page

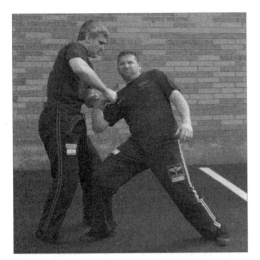

Figure 4.07e

Figures 4.07a–e. Using a sidestep body defense and simultaneous angled forearm block, deflect-redirect the weapon and launch simultaneous punches to the attacker's head. As learned with the instinctive defense, do not break contact with the weapon arm. The angled block creates a "V" with your arm overtop the attacking arm while securing the assailant's wrist. Your blocking arm targets just above the assailant's wrist where one would normally wear a wristwatch. Your counterstrikes should stun your assailant and allow you to press the counterattack. Keep in mind he will retract his stabbing arm.

After the block and simultaneous counterpunches are delivered, without breaking contact, secure the wrist while your counterattack arm now secures the hand for a Cavalier #1 weapon removal. You may add a simultaneous kick to the groin with the cavalier by performing a scissors kick (jumping on your kicking leg while pulling your non-kicking leg into your chest).

Note: For this defense—unlike the previous instinctive defense—do not counterattack using knee strikes because you can injure yourself with the blade you are pinning against the attacker's torso or hip.

Defending an Off-Angle Underhand Stab

An assailant may attempt to low stab you from an indirect angle.

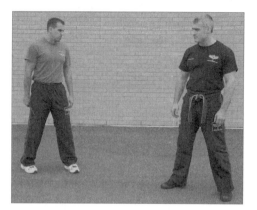

Figure 4.08a

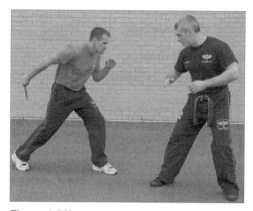

Figure 4.08b

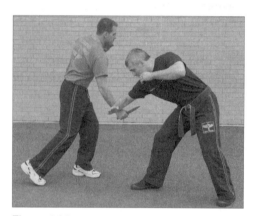

Figure 4.08c

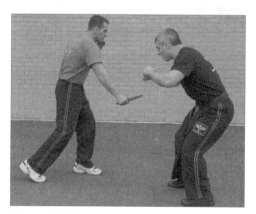

Figure 4.08d

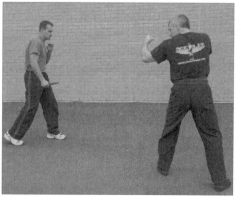

Figure 4.08e

Figures 4.08a–e. This type of attack, because of its short distance and rapidity, might require you to deflect-redirect the attack and immediately back away from the assailant using tsai-bake to either retreat or continue to defend against follow-on attack. This defense uses a horizontal block with the nearside arm (similar to the instinctive underhand stab) to redirect-deflect.

Defending an Off-Angle Straight Stab

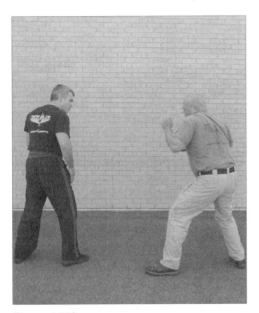

Figure 4.08f

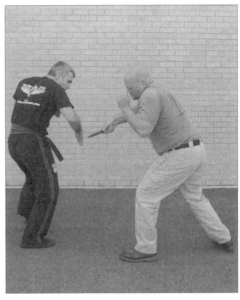

Figure 4.08g

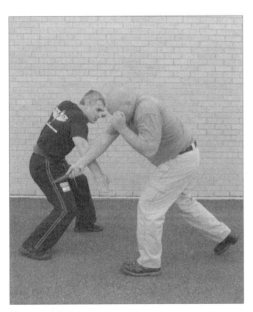

Figure 4.08h

Figures 4.08f–h. Against a low straight stab, step forward with your farside leg to move you off the line of attack while using your nearside hand to deflect the stab and quickly control the attacker's arm by knifing your arm down (similar to an overhead impact weapon deflection-redirection except here you are stabbing down), and immediately snake the deflecting-redirecting arm around the assailant's arm to secure the edged weapon. Note that this can be very difficult if the assailant retracts his arm.

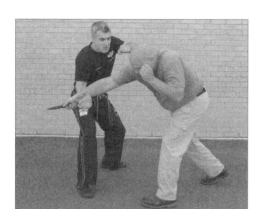

Figure 4.08i

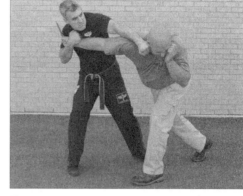

Figure 4.08j

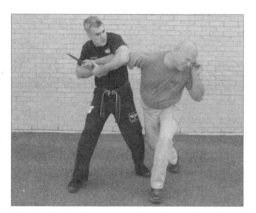

Figure 4.08k

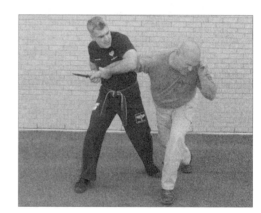

Figure 4.08l

Figures 4.08i–l. A simultaneous punch or eye gouge must be delivered with your outside arm. After snaking and taking control of the assailant's arm, additional retzev combatives are available, such as knee strikes, eye rakes, and neck cranks, or Cavalier #1. Again, be sure to stay behind the assailant and inside the arc of the edged weapon. The edged weapon may also be taken away by switching your control hands. In addition, Control Hold C may be applied to take the assailant down, forcing his arm forward and down just above his elbow. As noted, it may be more prudent, depending on your recognition and reaction time to block and move away from the strike, to either disengage or run away, or re-engage as appropriate.

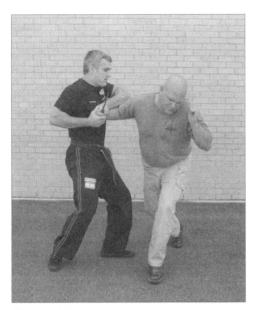

Figure 4.08m

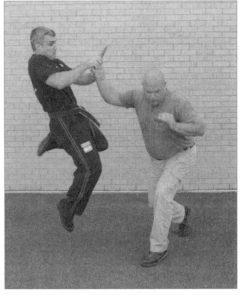

Figure 4.08n

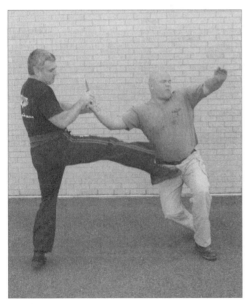

Figure 4.08o

Figures 4.08m–o. An advanced variation utilizes a jumping scissors kick to the opponent's groin while applying crushing wrist pressure to the opponent. To execute the kick properly, jump high on the kicking leg while pulling the non-kicking leg high into your chest to elevate the jump. (Both legs do not jump together.) Note that this disarming method with modification is used to take down an assailant threatening with a hand grenade.

Defending a Midsection Hook Stab or Slash

Another typical attack is a hook stab or slash to the midsection.

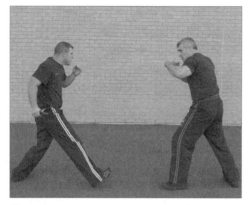

Figure 4.09a

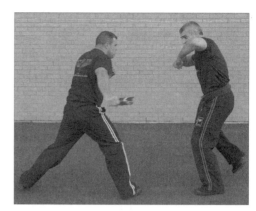

Figure 4.09b

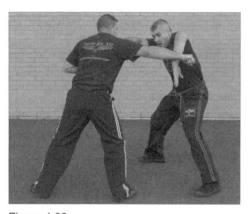

Figure 4.09c

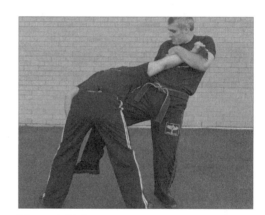

Figure 4.09d

Figures 4.09a–d. Similar to the overhead stab defense, use a body defense by stepping away from the edged-weapon's attack path while simultaneously blocking and counterstriking. Your blocking arm inverts to form an upside down "L" with fingers pointed toward the ground. Simultaneous counterstrikes can include punches to the face or strikes to the throat. As with the other edged-weapon defenses, contact is maintained with the assailant's arm as you once again snake the arm for control followed up with additional knee combatives. Once the assailant is debilitated, follow up with a Cavalier #2 or Control Hold A weapon removal options.

Defending an Inside Slash

Long Range Slash

An inside slash against the throat is one of the most common attacks. (Note, from a long range, you also might use a roundhouse kick against the slash as depicted in Figures 3.03g–h.)

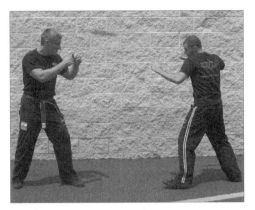

Figure 4.10a

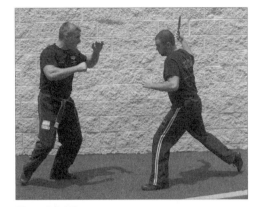

Figure 4.10b

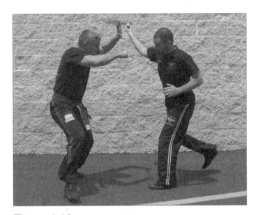

Figure 4.10c

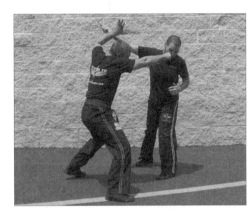

Figure 4.10d

Figures 4.10a–d. This defense, by design, is similar to the overhead attack defense depicted in Figures 4.01a–t. The assailant has the edged weapon in his right hand and is facing you. The defense once again involves a simultaneous three-part movement primarily relying on our instinct to block and step away from the inside slash. The step away is absolutely critical to defend against the inside slash, especially when the assailant uses a short slash keeping the elbow of his slashing arm close to his body. If the assailant used a hook stab and tried to burst directly, you would go directly into the point of the incoming knife (depicted in Figures 4.21a–c). If you directly burst in, you will be lacerated. Block the assailant's right edged-weapon hand using an outside block by rotating your left arm (nearest to the edged weapon) outside to deflect the assailant's right arm away from your head. Do not break contact to maintain control while simultaneously striking the assailant in the face or throat as you step diagonally forward with the outside right leg to take you off the line of attack. Block and stop the attack by rotating your left arm outward and then immediately rotating the arm back to grab and secure the assailant's right wrist and drive his edged-weapon arm back while delivering punishing knee strikes.

As emphasized when defending an overhead attack, it is paramount that you take a step away from the attack and then drive the assailant's arm back for control. Again, after stepping off the line of attack, driving the assailant's arm back serves two purposes: (1) it prevents the assailant from initiating further attacks, and (2) it positions you to apply strong control hold options. Remember that kravists train to use wrist releases; therefore, we know an assailant could use the same release against us. Wrist releases, when holding a blade, present special dangers because not only can the assailant release, but he can also slash and stab while doing it.

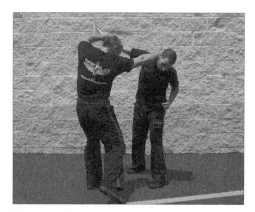

Figure 4.10e

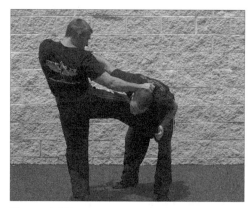

Figure 4.10f

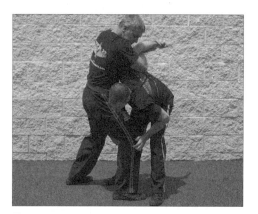

Figure 4.10g

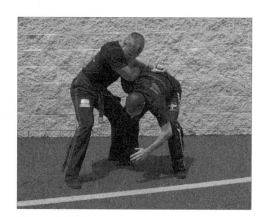

Figure 4.10h

Figures 4.10e–h. Control Hold A, as learned previously, powerfully secures the assailant driving him face-down—importantly, placing strong control over the edged-weapon hand. Control the edged weapon and remove it with precision from the assailant's grip. Use your left hand to remove it from the assailant's grip by securing the edged weapon at the bottom of the hilt, inserting your thumb, and prying it from the assailant's grip toward his head. Another option is to keep the assailant's elbow pinned to your body and slip your right hand out to pry the edged weapon away.

Medium Range Slash

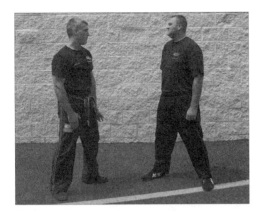

Figure 4.10i

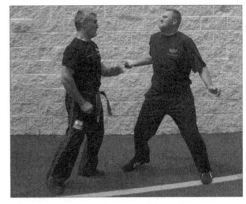

Figure 4.10j

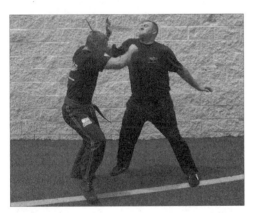

Figure 4.10k

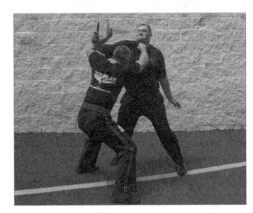

Figure 4.10l

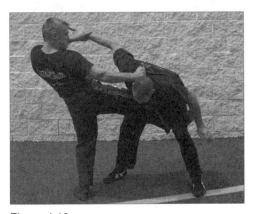

Figure 4.10m

Figures 4.10i–m. From a medium-close range, you must once again use the quickest intercept-block by stepping off the line of attack combined with a simultaneous straight punch. Immediately transition to control the weapon arm and proceed with retzev combatives and your preferred disarm including Control Hold A or Cavalier #2.

Short Range Slash

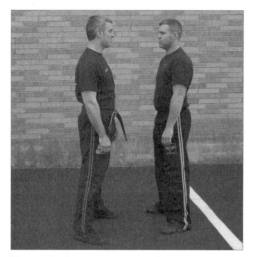

Figure 4.10n

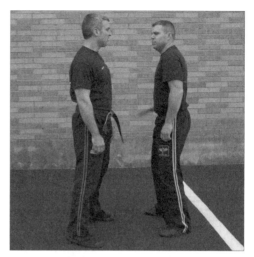

Figure 4.10o

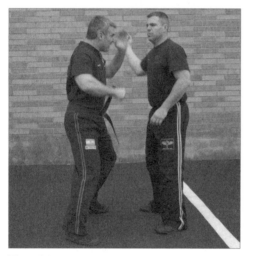

Figure 4.10p

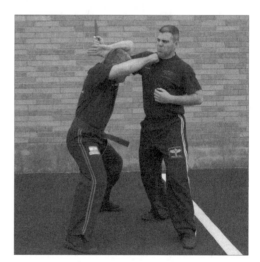

Figure 4.10q

Figures 4.10n–q. From an extreme-close range, you must use the quickest intercept-block, which is an angled gun block combined with a simultaneous straight punch. Immediately transition to control the weapon arm and proceed with retzev combatives and your preferred disarm including Control Hold A or Cavalier #2.

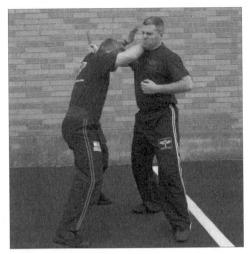

Figure 4.10r

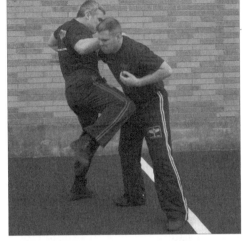

Figure 4.10s

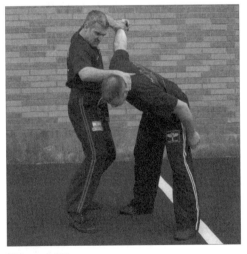

Figure 4.10t

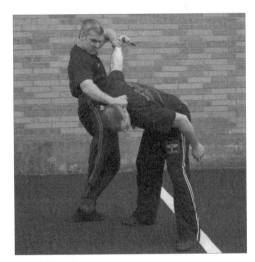

Figure 4.10u

Figures 4.10r–u. Continue with knee combatives to the midsection. If you drop his level, a knee strike to his head can end the confrontation quickly.

An add-on option to defend the attack uses the primary defense to block-sidestep and attack method, but follows up with a debilitating straight left kick to the assailant's groin rather attempting to control the attacking arm as depicted in Fkgures 4.01l–s. Remember, the sidestep has placed the right leg forward to take you off the line of attack. Your weight has shifted to your left leg positioning you to deliver a debilitating left straight kick to the assailant's groin and then to quickly disengage while continuing to break the angle (moving away from the edged weapon). This option also allows you to deploy a firearm or impact weapon if available.

As noted previously, a specific third law-enforcement option is to complete the block-sidestep counterattack and then immediately draw to instinctively point shoot the assailant. Note again, blocking and simultaneously drawing the weapon is not an optimum tactic because the assailant is coming at you full speed and force, likely with repeated stabs and you have not stunned him. Instead, you are relying on your ability to deploy and successfully use your weapon, which, unfortunately, has had fatal consequences for many police and security officers. You should continue to move away from the edged-weapon arm. In short, this defense can be combined with an initial strike to momentarily stun the assailant, create distance, and deploy a firearm.

A fourth option is to use a body defense retreat while covering your throat and face by rotating your arms so that the backs of your hands face the assailant to protect your arteries. The closer the assailant is to you, the more difficult it will be for you to use a body-defense retreat. You have a farther distance to pull yourself back out of harm's way. As the slash comes toward your head, lift your front heel slightly off the ground to momentarily perch on the ball of your foot, which will shift your weight back slightly. Simultaneously retract your arms in from your regular outlet stance to form a defensive shield in front of your throat with your forearms out to the side and your palm heels resting on the crown of your skull. As the weapon continues its horizontal arc and passes your covering arms, immediately burst inside while rotating your arms outward to trap the edged-weapon arm while delivering simultaneous combatives. This defense is described in the next technique, depicted in Figures 4.11.

Defending an Inside Diagonal Slash

This defense, by design, is similar to both the overhead attack and inside slash defenses. The assailant has the edged weapon in his right hand and is facing you. This defense once again involves a simultaneous three-part movement, with a strong emphasis on stepping off the line to get inside the arc of the edged weapon. The defense again relies on your instinct to block and step away from the inside slash. As noted, the step away is absolutely critical to defend against the diagonal inside slash, especially when the assailant uses a short slash keeping the elbow of his slashing arm close to his body. If you burst directly in, you will be lacerated. Block the assailant's right edged weapon hand using an outside block by rotating your left arm (nearest to the edged weapon) outside to deflect the assailant's right arm away from your head. Do not break contact to maintain control while simultaneously striking the assailant in the face or throat as you step diagonally forward with the outside right leg to take you off the line of attack. In other words, block the attack by rotating your left arm outward and then immediately rotating the arm back to grab and secure the assailant's right wrist and drive his edged-weapon arm back while delivering punishing knee strikes. Follow the same removal as described in the previous figures in series 4.10.

Body Defense an Inside Forward Slash and Follow-up Backslash

If an assailant misses with an inside slash, a natural follow-up attack is to bring the blade back across your throat or face using an outside slash.

When the defender uses correct timing to avoid the initial attack with the forward slash missing its mark, a backslash usually follows as the assailant continues to press his attack. In other words, you must with correct timing retreat and then immediately burst back in with decisive counterattacks to stop the attack. This can be a difficult technique to execute, especially against an assailant using short or tight slashes (which is why leg defenses against edged-weapon attacks to your torso and head can be so effective).

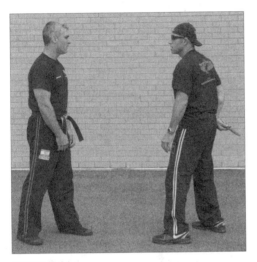

Figure 4.11a

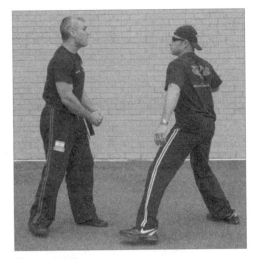

Figure 4.11b

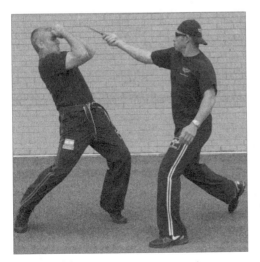

Figure 4.11c

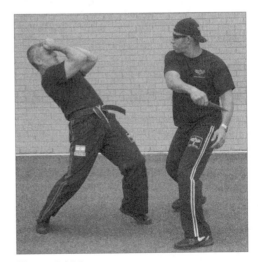

Figure 4.11d

Figures 4.11a–d. Use an upper body retreat defense by bringing your hands close to your face to protect your throat. Turn your hands palm in to protect the arteries in your arm. Your bodyweight must transfer backward to remove your torso from harm's way. You have a choice to rise onto the ball of the foot of your lead leg, or to keep the front foot planted. This foot movement will depend on your weight distribution at the time of the defense. If you were preparing to kick with your front leg, the weight is on your rear leg, and you will find it easier to rise onto the ball of the front leg. Conversely, if your weight is forward on your front leg, rising onto the ball of your foot may not feel as natural and you may wish to simply transfer your weight back.

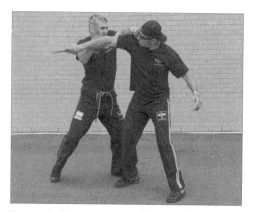

Figure 4.11e

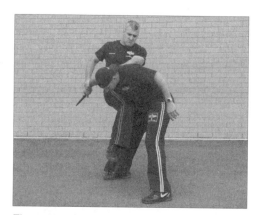

Figure 4.11f

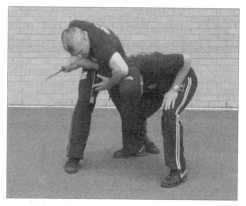

Figure 4.11g

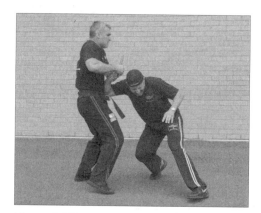

Figure 4.11h

Figures 4.11e–h. Once the assailant's forward slash has passed you, with good footwork, immediately burst into the assailant with the bony side (ulna) of both of your forearms and inverted punch over the top of the attacker's slashing arm. Be sure to use an inverted punch to drive his aim down. Remove the weapon using Cavalier #1.

The goal is to burst inside the backslash arc of the edged weapon and jam the assailant's edged-weapon arm. Block and trap the assailant's arm while executing a near-simultaneous sliding over the top counterpunch with your inside arm to the attacker's head. Be aware that this bursting forward with all of your bodyweight is likely to drive the attacker backward, but do not lose contact with the attacker's edged-weapon arm. Contact provides you with the ability to exert end control over the weapon and, ultimately, the attacker. Immediately use your other arm to secure the wrist and establish control over the assailant's edged-weapon arm to allow for debilitating knee strikes. Another control option is to snake your blocking arm immediately underneath and around the assailant's edged-weapon forearm, and either fishhook his eye or reach around to control his chin and rotate him decisively to the ground with an one-hundred-eighty-degree (tsai-bake) step. Be sure to maintain firm control of the edged-weapon arm and keep it away from your neck and head staying inside and clear of the edged-weapon's dangerous arc. You have several options to remove the edged weapon including Cavalier #1, or Control Hold C, or torquing the assailant's neck with your free arm to take him down for additional combatives. Be sure to stay inside the edged-weapon's arc and keep it away from your throat. Another option is to shatter the assailant's elbow using your forearm or a sharp palm heel, however, the assailant will drop the edged weapon, which could present a danger to you should an unfriendly third party pick it up.

Note: This defense would be the same using a baton or even another edged weapon against a backslash using different counterattacks and weapon disarms.

Backslash Defense or Against a "Reverse" Stab

As examined in the previous defense against an inside and follow-up outside slash, this defense requires the defender to close the distance against the assailant to stop his edged-weapon wielding arm, using a double-handed forearm block and sliding punch to thwart the attack. This defense is depicted in Figures 4.11e–h.

The goal is to burst forward once again inside the backslash arc to jam the assailant's edged-weapon arm. Block and trap the assailant's arm while executing a near-simultaneous sliding over-the-top counterpunch with your inside arm to the attacker's head. Be aware that bursting forward with all of your bodyweight may drive the attacker backward, but again do not lose contact with the attacker's edged-weapon arm. Contact provides you with the ability to exert control to disable the assailant and take away the weapon. Immediately use your other arm to secure the wrist and establish control over the assailant's edged-weapon arm to allow for debilitating knee strikes. Another option is to snake your blocking arm immediately underneath and around the assailant's edged-weapon forearm, and either fishhook his eye or reach around to control his chin and rotate him decisively to the ground with a one-hundred-eighty-degree (tsai-bake) step. Be sure to maintain firm control of the edged-weapon arm, and keep it away from your neck and head while staying inside and clear of the edged-weapon's dangerous arc. You have several options to remove the edged weapon including Cavalier #1, or Control Hold C, or torquing the assailant's neck with your free arm to take him down for additional combatives. Be sure to stay inside the edged-weapon's arc and keep it away from your throat. Another option is to shatter the assailant's elbow using your forearm or a sharp palm heel; however, the assailant will drop the edged weapon, which could present a danger to you should an unfriendly third party pick it up.

Note: This defense would be the same using a baton or even another edged weapon against a backslash using different counterattacks and weapon disarms.

Body Defense Against a Backslash and Follow-up Inside Slash

If an assailant misses with an outside slash, a natural follow-up attack is to bring the blade back across your throat or face using an inside slash.

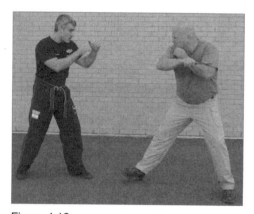

Figure 4.12a

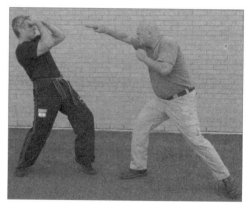

Figure 4.12b

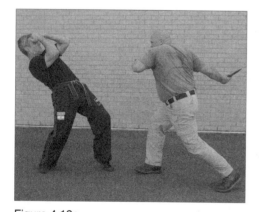

Figure 4.12c

Figures 4.12a–d. Caption on next page

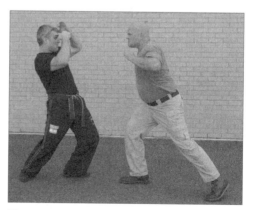

Figure 4.12d

Figures 4.12a–d. A backslash that missed its mark is easily followed by a forward slash. Retreat, and then immediately burst with a stop to the outside using inside decisive counterattacks to stop the attack. Your bodyweight must transfer backward to remove your torso from harm's way. You have a choice to rise onto the ball of the foot of your lead leg, or to keep the front foot planted. This foot movement will depend on your weight distribution at the time of the defense. If you were preparing to kick with your front leg, hence, the weight is on your rear leg, and you will find it easier to rise onto the ball of the front leg. Conversely, if your weight is forward on your front leg, rising onto the ball of your foot may not feel as natural and you may wish to simply transfer your weight back. Again, this can be a difficult technique to execute, especially against an assailant using short or tight slashes, so your timing must be excellent and finish as you would against a front slash.

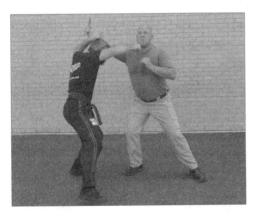

Figure 4.12e

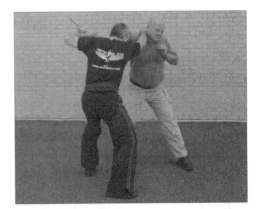

Figure 4.12f

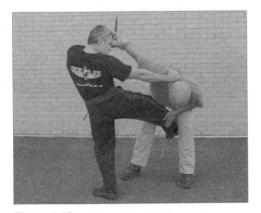

Figure 4.12g

Figures 4.12e–g. Complete the defense, as you would defend against a basic inside slash as in Figures 4.10, using whichever control hold and weapon removal technique you most prefer.

Defending a Stab or Slash to the Legs

An assailant may decide to target your legs, particularly, your femoral artery or groin.

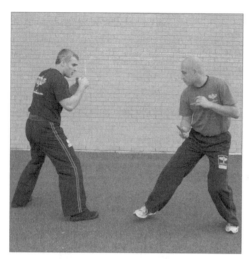

Figure 4.13a

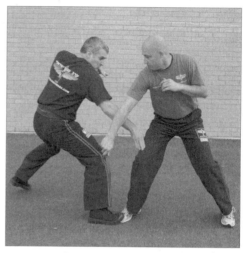

Figure 4.13b

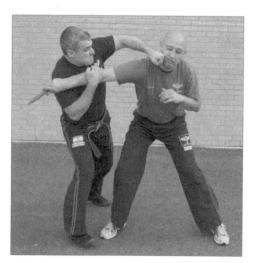

Figure 4.13c

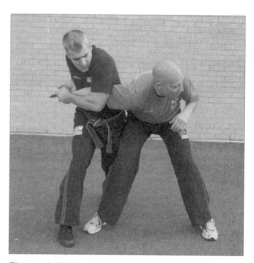

Figure 4.13d

Figures 4.13a–d. Defending against edged-weapon attacks to the legs is challenging. You must drop your level to the assailant's level to prepare for the defense. If the assailant is in a crouch, you too, must crouch. When defending against a straight stab or slash to the groin or legs, krav maga uses the same defenses you have learned in Figures 4.08f–o.

Note that your balance and weight transfer will change as you lower your center of gravity. Practice and feel comfortable with this. You may also use body defenses to avoid the initial attacks and then, with correct timing, kick the assailant in the head but this is risky because he can easily stab or slash your legs. An alternate option is to use a body defense sliding your legs back out of the edged-weapon's arc, and then close with an arm defense to control the weapon and debilitate the assailant.

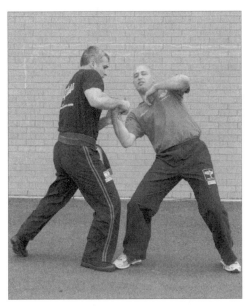 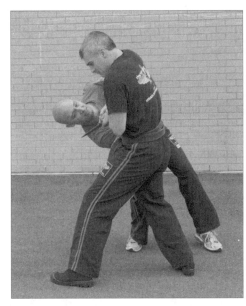

Figure 4.13e   Figure 4.13f

Figures 4.13e–f. Complete the defense using Cavalier #1 or Head Control to remove the weapon.

Defending an Assailant Who Strikes/Kicks and Stabs/Slashes

An assailant might punch, kick, or otherwise use his free hand to attack you followed immediately by an edged-weapon attack.

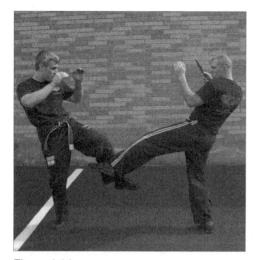

Figure 4.14a

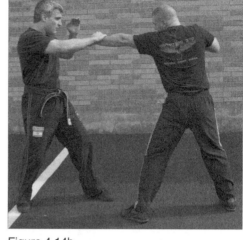

Figure 4.14b

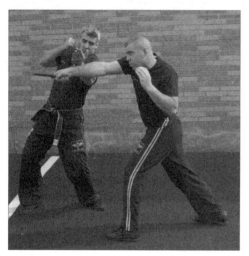

Figure 4.14c

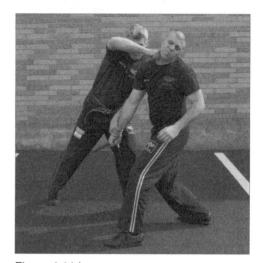

Figure 4.14d

Figures 4.14a–d. Defend against all strikes while keeping your focus on the weapon. His strikes can hurt you; his weapon can kill you. In this instance, defend the kick, punch, and straight stab seriatim making sure to step off the line of attack. Nevertheless, the assailant's strikes can set you up for disaster. Your defenses must account for the entire attack. As always in a weapons defense, maim or stun your opponent, and close in on the edged weapon to secure it as soon as possible. Complete the defense using Cavalier #1.

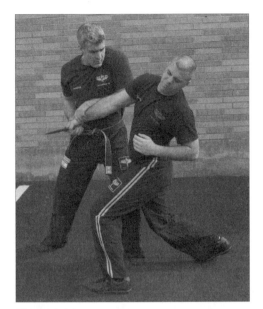 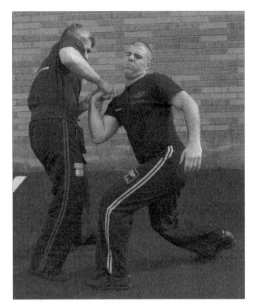

Figure 4.14e   Figure 4.14f

Figures 4.14e–f. Continue the defense and remove the weapon using Cavalier #1.

The IKMA's yellow, orange, and green belts develop the core methods to defend against unarmed assaults, particularly, by developing knock-out/down power. These levels also incorporate some of the basic defenses against edged-weapon assaults while focusing on unarmed combatives such as straight punches and kicks.

Defending Continuous Edged-Weapon Attacks

The assailant may try more than one attack with the weapon and often vary the angle or method of slashes or stabs. Of course, to preempt this continuous attack cycle, try to stun the assailant with counterattacks in the first place. While not optimum, it may be that you need to counterattack and retreat only to re-engage again to finally close on the assailant to disarm him. It is paramount to use correct timing. This situation also demonstrates why krav maga emphasizes strong punishing combatives, not breaking contact with the edged-weapon arm after the deflection-redirection, and securing the edged-weapon arm immediately while simultaneously debilitating the assailant.

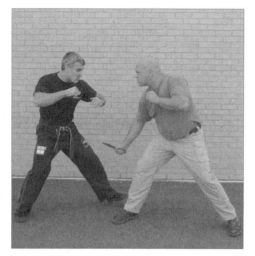

Figure 4.15a

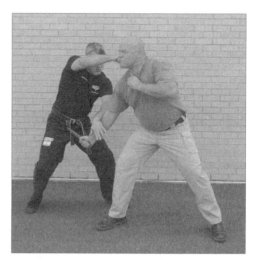

Figure 4.15b

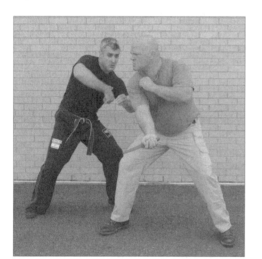

Figure 4.15c

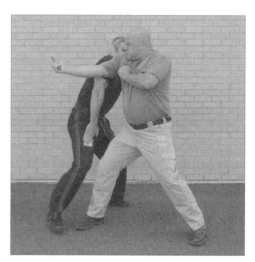

Figure 4.15d

Figures 4.15a–d. The key is to remain either off the line of attack or jam the arm to seize dominant control as soon as possible. The photos show one particular stab pattern of an underneath stab, a hook stab, and then a stab at the defender's neck. The initial deflection-redirection is the same as learned previously against a recognized underhand stab; however, the assailant successfully retracts the edged weapon. Continue to move deep into the deadside keeping the nearside arm pointed down and flush against your torso. Bring the opposite hand, palm in, up to your throat with fingers

Figures 4.15a–d. Caption continue on next page

pointed upward flush to your body with the palm turned toward your head to protect your vital arteries. This combination arm-work allows you to jam the assailant's movements and quickly pincer his weapon arm with your underneath arm to control it. Pin the assailant's forearm tight against your body to prevent or limit any arm movement to protect yourself from the blade. This is best done by securing your front forearm in the crook of his elbow fulcrum and your rear arm against his wrist. Simultaneously, rake his eyes with your other arm. You may also pincer both arms around his weapon arm and deliver knee attacks to his thigh. As with all defenses, be sure to maintain strict control of the edged-weapon arm, especially important when the edged weapon is held high near your head and throat. Use Cavalier #1. This example includes a modified roundhouse kick sweep to the assailant's Achilles. Again, be sure to control the edged weapon safely.

There are a wide variety of these dangerous slash and stab attack options. The best advice to keep in mind if you cannot control the weapon with your initial defense is to follow or defend against the most logical attack patterns or natural progression of the edged weapon after it is blocked. As always, secure the edged weapon as soon as possible while initiating the most direct opportunistic counterattacks.

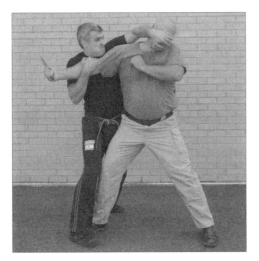

Figure 4.15e

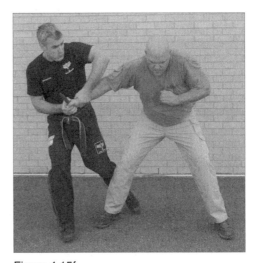

Figure 4.15f

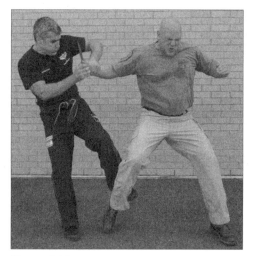

Figure 4.15g

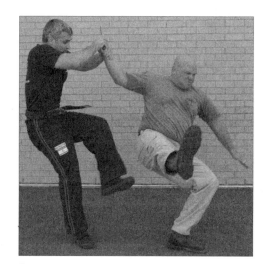

Figure 4.15h

Figures 4.15e–h. Complete the defense using Cavalier #1. One variation is to sweep the attacker's nearside leg to take him down hard. Be sure to have strict control of the weapon.

Late Defense Using Minimum Deflection-Redirection and Tsai-bake

An attacker may catch you completely off-guard and you may only be able to step away from the attack with a minimal deflection-redirection.

If an attacker armed with an edged weapon begins his arm motion against you, you may only have time to instinctively shield yourself with your nearside arm. Unlike the previous defenses where because of your recognition, you are able to tense the deflection-redirection arm and forcefully engage the attacking arm. You are simply slapping the weapon arm away while moving off the line of attack. As with all krav maga defenses, you must counterattack. You can use a palm-heel or knuckles strike to the attacker's nearside ear. Similar to previous defenses, the counterattack and footwork are in concert. The counterattack must be quick. The one-hundred-eighty-degree (tsai-bake) step is vital to moving away from the attack and allowing you to retreat. You may continue to retreat, or if the assailant continues the attack, engage with the appropriate technique.

Defense Against an Assailant Who Engages You in Conversation Hiding the Weapon and Then Attacks

An assailant might first converse with you as a distraction or somehow lure you into lowering your defenses. As always, awareness training is most important. If you do not know someone, watch his or her hand movements. You are perfectly within your rights to demand that someone show you his or her hands. If you are convinced an attack is imminent, distract and kick the suspected assailant in the groin or knee, and then close to subdue the threat. After the kick(s), you may also simply run. If the person was reaching into his back pocket or waistband to pull out a weapon, you were justified. If he or she is reaching for an innocuous object such as a cell phone, you will have to give a very sincere, perhaps costly apology.

Defense Against an Assailant Who First Engages You in an Unarmed Fight and Then Attacks With an Edged Weapon

You could find yourself caught in a violent encounter with someone who mid-fight decides to pull an edged weapon out on you. Often this happens when an assailant is on the losing end of an unarmed confrontation. Again, awareness training is crucial. Equally important, krav maga emphasizes neutralizing the opponent in the first place through decisive combatives or control holds. If, however, the opponent pulls out a weapon, keep the momentum on your side while recognizing—even if you did not previously—that the attack is now a life and death matter. However, it is wise to always consider a violent attack a potential life and death situation.

Edged-Weapon Threats

We hope your awareness and preemptive capabilities would never allow the following scenarios to happen. In other words, you would recognize and interdict the threat before he can present a weapon much less close on you to hold an edged weapon to your throat. Nevertheless, krav maga deals with worst-case scenarios such as when an assailant catches you unaware, for example, placing an edged weapon to your throat or back.

Edged-Weapon Threats against Your Throat
An assailant can hold an edged weapon to your throat and threaten in two typical situations: (1) the edged weapon is held to throat with the assailant's palm facing up, or (2) it is held across the throat with the assailant's palm down. In either case, the assailant might also grab you with his other arm.

If you recognize the threat prior to the assailant placing the blade to your throat, you could use a lowline kick targeting the assailant's groin or knees. If the assailant has closed on you but not yet brought the weapon to your throat because he is in process, you could use the outside slash defense covered in Figures 4.10a–m.

If the assailant succeeds in surprising you by placing the weapon against your throat, you must move your head back to clear the weapon from your throat while simultaneously yanking the assailant's edged-weapon arm down and away from your throat.

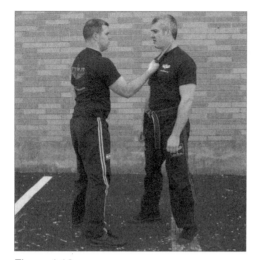

Figure 4.16a

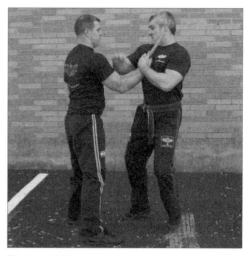

Figure 4.16b

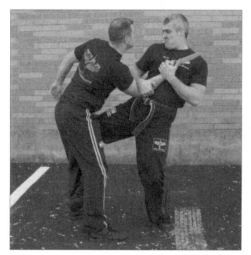

Figure 4.16c

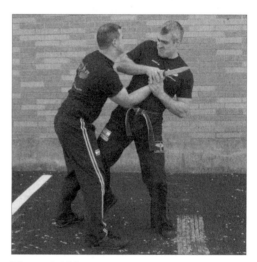

Figure 4.16d

Figures 4.16a–d. To redirect-deflect the weapon, yank down on the assailant's knuckles to pin his wrist to your body while moving your head back to also clear the blade. Clasp the attacker's hand at the knuckles while pivoting your body away from the assailant. As you pluck with your nearside hand, simultaneously secure the weapon with your other hand so that both of your arms are clamped down on his arms. As you secure the attacker's wrist by pinning it to your chest and pivoting, simultaneously secure his edged-weaponarm by wrapping your opposite arm around it while delivering a straight knee to the groin with your nearside leg.

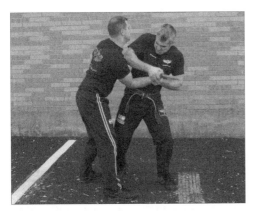

Figure 4.16e

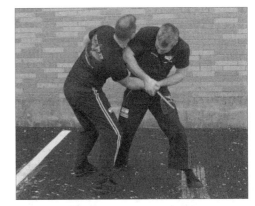

Figure 4.16f

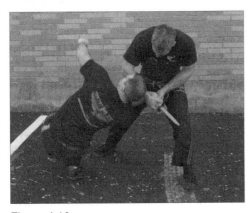

Figure 4.16g

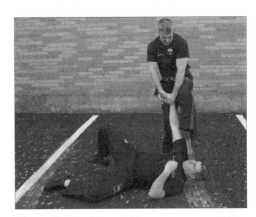

Figure 4.16h

Figures 4.16e–h. Continue the defense with multiple knee strikes and then a modified Cavalier #1. Note: The assailant might also grab you with his other arm. The defense remains the same except you must concentrate on pinning his edged-weapon wielding arm.

A variation is if the assailant holds the weapon across your throat with his palm down. Again, if you recognize the threat prior to the assailant placing the blade to your throat, you could use a lowline kick targeting the assailant's groin or knees. If the assailant has closed on you but not brought the weapon to your throat because he is in process, you could use the L block defense covered in Figures 4.04a–m. Should the assailant succeed in surprising you by placing the weapon against your throat with his other hand on your torso, move your head back using a body defense to clear your throat and deflect the assailant's edged-weapon arm away.

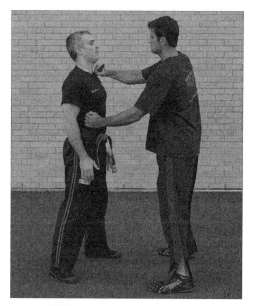

Figure 4.17a

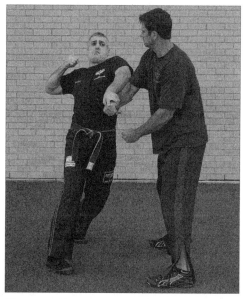

Figure 4.17b

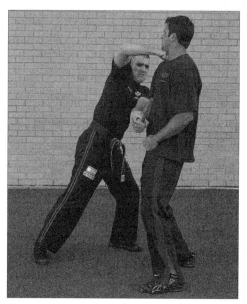

Figure 4.17c

Figures 4.17a–c. If the assailant threatens you while gripping the edged weapon with his palm down across your throat, execute a simultaneous deflection-redirection and body defense to clear the edged weapon from your throat with simultaneous counterstrikes to his head. As you deflect the edged weapon from your throat, secure the arm by bracing your forearm on a slight angle against the threat arm using an elbow kiss. Pin his arm to his body to protect against a backslash or other offensive movement. Press the counterattack, secure the arm, and take him down with a cavalier.

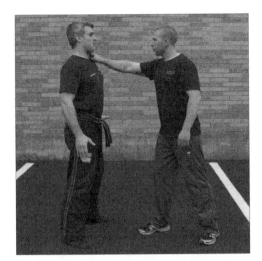

Figure 4.17d

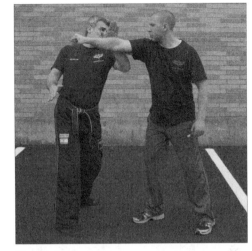

Figure 4.17e

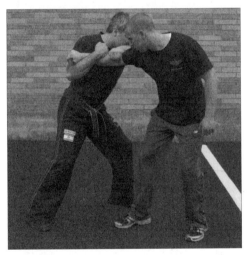

Figure 4.17f

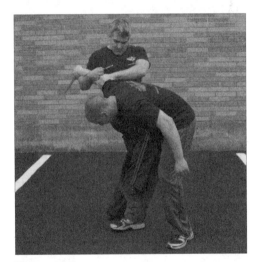

Figure 4.17g

Figures 4.17d–g. You may also use two arms to deflect-redirect the weapon by using the palm of your nearside hand. As you deflect with your nearside hand, simultaneously bring your opposite arm up to secure the weapon with your other hand so that both of your arms are clamped down on his. Note that this defense is used when he is not securing you with his other arm. Essentially, you are deflecting his arm into your other arm while catching his weapon arm in the process.

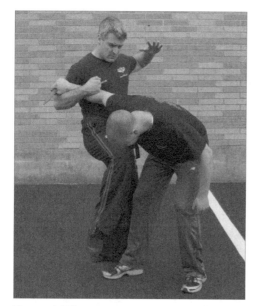

Figure 4.17h

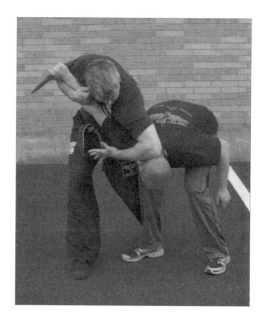

Figure 4.17i

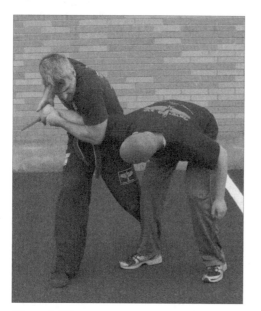

Figure 4.17j

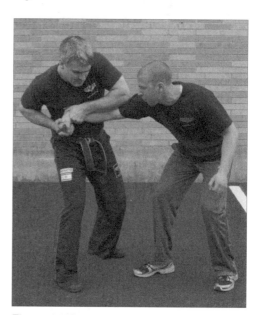

Figure 4.17k

Figures 4.17h–k. As you secure the attacker's wrist by pinning it to your chest with both arms, deliver a straight knee to the groin with your nearside leg. Continue the defense with multiple knee strikes, elbow strikes, and then a Cavalier #1.

If the threat were to come from one hand with the edged-weapon tip pointing up underneath your chin, yank down on the assailant's hand just below to thumb joint to exert great pressure on the wrist while simultaneously embedding your thumb into the assailant's eye socket followed by a swift knee strike to the groin. You could also use an uppercut punch. If the assailant grabs you with two arms, you may still use the eye gouge or a knee strike to the groin. If you use the knee strike as your initial counterattack, be sure to use both of your arms to control the assailant's weapon arm by using your non-plucking hand to exert Cavalier #1. Note: The control over the edged-weapon hand is a partial-cavalier. As you press the counterattack and the assailant has been suitably "softened up," use a full Cavalier #1 to take him down.

Edged-Weapon Threat to Your Back

A threat, particularly an armed robbery attempt, might come from the rear if the assailant seeks to take you by surprise. This defense deflects the edged weapon away with control combined with an immediate counterstrike. (Note that a gun threat from the rear is the same except for the weapon removal.)

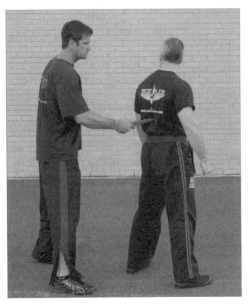

Figure 4.18a

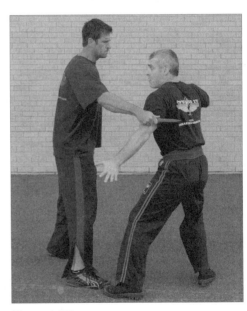

Figure 4.18b

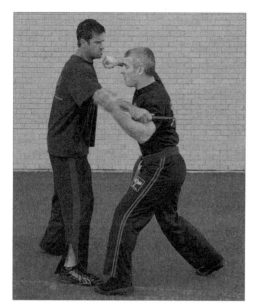

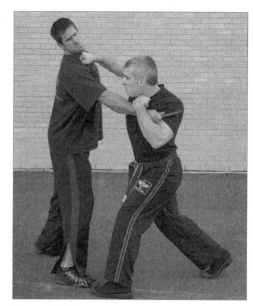

Figure 4.18c

Figure 4.18d

Figures 4.18a–d. To defend, you must turn your head to recognize and assess any threat from the rear. In other words, the head always leads the body. Redirect the edged threat by turning into the assailant with your left arm and deflecting-redirecting the assailant's weapon arm away with the upper part of your left forearm, which immediately snakes around the weapon arm. Take a direct step—not a looping step—to close the distance to the assailant. As you secure the assailant's arm, simultaneously counterattack with a punch or other strike to the head or throat. Note that when turning into the assailant, do not use an elbow strike because it is a short strike. You must always be able to reach the assailant, especially when there is a large height or reach disparity. In addition, an elbow strike requires you to move your control farther up the weapon arm preventing you from controlling the weapon arm's wrist.

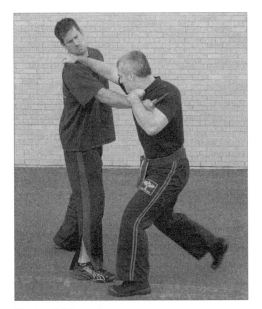

Figure 4.18e

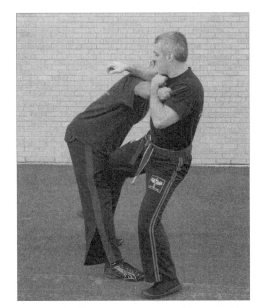

Figure 4.18f

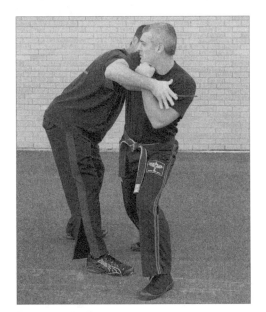

Figure 4.18g

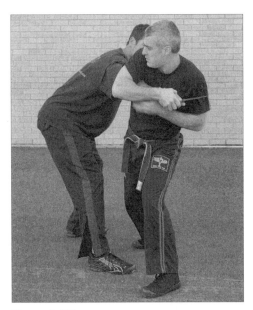

Figure 4.18h

Figures 4.18e–h. Control and disarm the assailant using Cavalier #2.

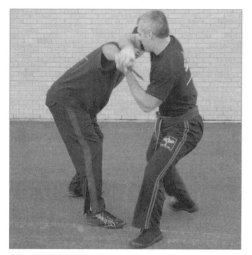

Figure 4.18i

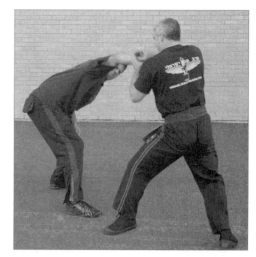

Figure 4.18j

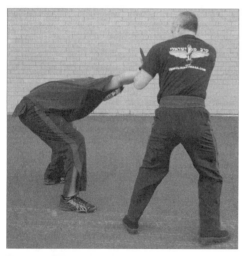

Figure 4.18k

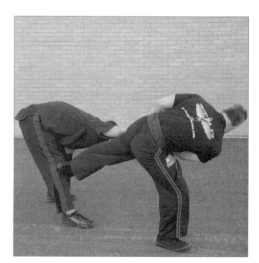

Figure 4.18l

Figures 4.18i–l. Turn decisively maintaining strict control of the weapon keeping it away from you by keeping your elbows close to your body. You may finish the technique with a sidekick to his nearside knee.

Edged-Weapon Threat to Your Throat from the Rear

This is an extremely dangerous situation because the assailant has considerable control over your body movement.

The defense against this type of threat to the rear is similar to the krav maga defense used against a rear choke; however, there is little margin for error. The weapon hand must be completely controlled.

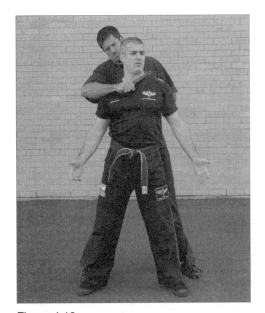

Figure 4.19a

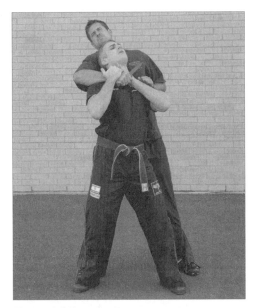

Figure 4.19b

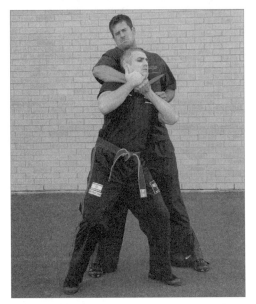

Figure 4.19c

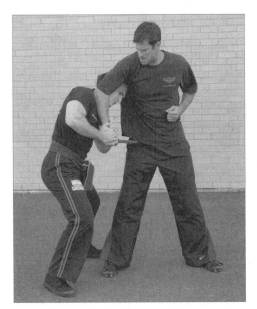

Figure 4.19d

Figures 4.19a–d. Clamp down on the assailant's arm with your farside arm and your hand closest to the edged weapon while delivering a simultaneous rear head-butt to the assailant's chin or nose. Slide your palmside arm out to help control the assailant's hand to exert maximum pressure and turn the edge away from your throat.

This control hold affords you tight control of the edged-weapon arm. Pull down forcefully with your farside arm and push down with your nearside hand. Tuck your chin to protect your throat and turn your left shoulder away from the blade. Clear the arm forcefully from your chin/neck area with your near hand while inserting your farside hand between the blade and your throat. Optimally, you will create a barrier with your hand, allowing you to push the threat away and assert control.

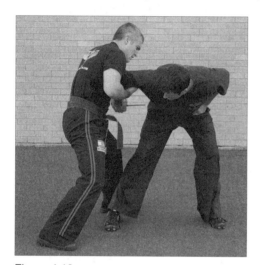

Figure 4.19e

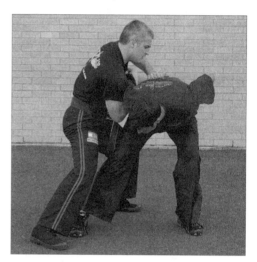

Figure 4.19f

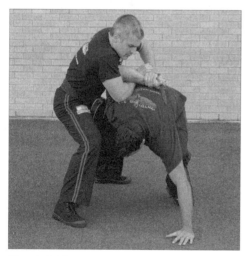

Figure 4.19g

Figures 4.19e–g. Dip your left shoulder and step backward with your left leg while wheeling your right shoulder in the direction of your assailant's right shoulder. Continue to step back underneath the assailant's right armpit while holding the assailant's arm firmly pinned against your body with both of your arms. Maintain strict control of the weapon. Keep his elbow compressed against your body, his weapon arm against your body to exert Police Control A, and/or knees to the midsection and thigh to collapse him. If the circumstances warrant, the edged weapon can be turned and used against the assailant.

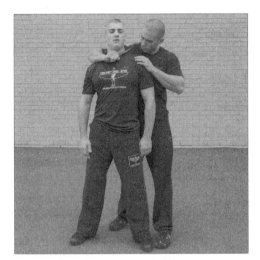

Figure 4.19h

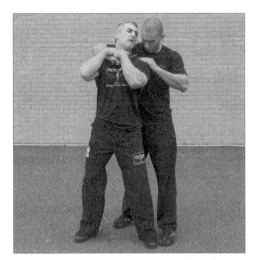

Figure 4.19i

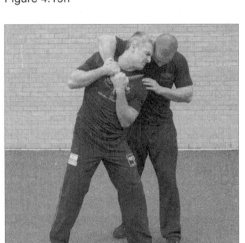

Figure 4.19j

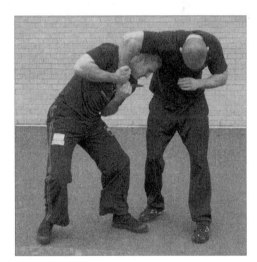

Figure 4.19k

Figures 4.19h–k. If the blade is touching your throat, and you feel you cannot insert your farside hand, you may yank down with both hands using all of your bodyweight to clear the edged weapon. Deliver a simultaneous head-butt to his temple. Dip your left shoulder and step backward with your left leg while wheeling your right shoulder in the direction of your assailant's right shoulder.

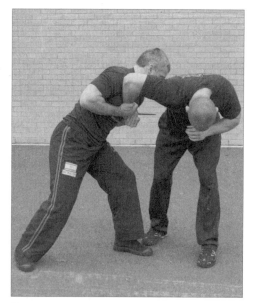

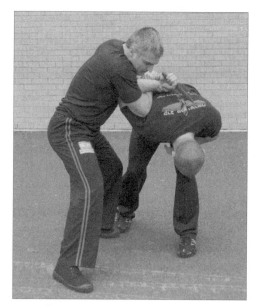

Figure 4.19l   Figure 4.19m

Figures 4.19l–m. Continue to step through and underneath the assailant's right armpit while holding the assailant's arm firmly pinned against your body with both of your arms. Press his weapon arm against your body to exert Police Control A and/or deliver knees to his midsection and nearside thigh to collapse him. Of course, if the circumstances warrant, the edged weapon can be turned and used against the assailant.

A third option in a worst-case scenario is to yank down with your nearside left hand to clasp the blade. Obviously, this will lacerate your hand, but the priority is to redirect the edged weapon away from your throat. As with all of these options, as soon as you create separation, dip your left shoulder and step backward with your left leg while wheeling your right shoulder in the direction of your assailant's right shoulder. Continue to step through and underneath the assailant's right armpit while holding the assailant's arm firmly pinned against your body with both of your arms resolutely controlling the assailant's edged-weapon arm. Immediately deliver a knee strike from your rear leg to the assailant's exposed midsection followed by additional retzev counterattacks into Control Hold A (Figures 4.19e–f). If necessary, you can also impale the assailant with his own weapon.

Edged-Weapon Threat from the Side behind the Arm

This is the same defense as an edged-weapon threat from the rear (Figures 4.18 series) but your turning radius is shorter.

Defenses When Both Combatants Are on the Ground

As noted in Chapter 3, you could find yourself in an unarmed groundfight and have it rapidly escalate into an edged-weapon attack. An open-handed groundfight can quickly escalate into a deadly struggle if one combatant produces an edged weapon. The defensive principles remain the same: you must deflect-redirect, use a body defense when possible, and counterattack simultaneously and relentlessly. As in a standing fight, there is a strong possibility that you may not realize the fight has instantaneously changed from an unarmed confrontation into an armed attack. Attacking your opponent's vital anatomy in any kind of combat is paramount. Striking the assailant in the eyes, throat, and groin may preempt his ability to deploy a weapon, especially when he is reaching for it. There are several places an assailant might hide a weapon including the small of his back, his waistband, his boot or sock, or his sleeve among other places.

Overhead Attack Defense with the Defender on His Back

When the defender is on his back and the assailant is on his knees, the preferred krav maga position (in any groundfight when the defender has his back to the ground) is to use a diagonal knee brace across the assailant's chest with your opposite foot on the assailant's sameside hip. Recall, as covered in Figures 3.11a–d, if you are on your back and the assailant deploys an edged weapon, a highly effective defense is to place your nearside foot on his edged-weapon wielding shoulder.

From your diagonal knee-brace position, you can defend an overhead attack similar to the standing off-angle overhead attack by using a body defense moving to the side combined with an outside deflection-redirection covered in Figures 4.03a–h. The defense against a right-handed overhead stab uses an outside block and body defense moving onto your right hip. This defensive movement brings you to the assailant's deadside allowing for multiple punches to the assailant's kidneys, armbars, or a rearmount.

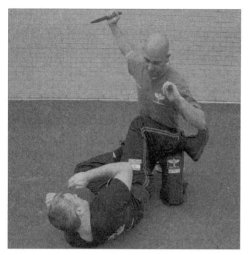

Figure 4.20a

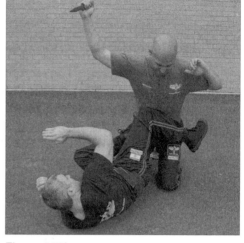

Figure 4.20b

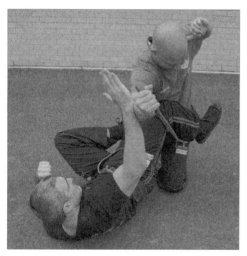

Figure 4.20c

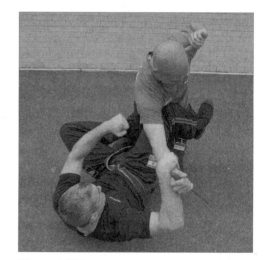

Figure 4.20d

Figures 4.20a–d. Block the assailant's right edged-weapon hand using an outside block by rotating your right arm (nearest to the edged weapon because of your body slide to the left) outside to deflect the assailant's right arm away from your head while punching him repeatedly in the kidneys. In short, the defense relies on your instinct to block and move away from a blow or stab.

Deflect the edged weapon as close as possible to the assailant's wrist.

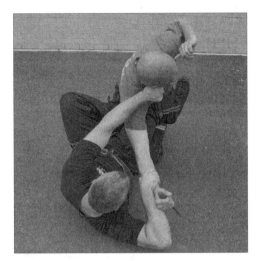

Figure 4.20e

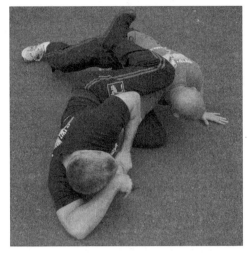

Figure 4.20f

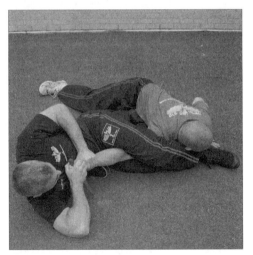

Figure 4.20g

Figures 4.20e–g. After striking the assailant in the head or the kidneys, press the counterattack by transitioning immediately from the block to securing that assailant's arm. Again, this maneuver is done by not breaking contact with the assailant's arm following the initial block. Try to maintain a grip on the assailant's arm with your deflecting-redirecting arm as you counterpunch him in the head. You can apply a face-down armbar to snap the assailant's arm making sure to maintain strict control of the edged weapon.

You might also be able to secure the arm with your blocking arm by turning on your side to smash or dislocate the assailant's elbow using a sharp forward blow just above the elbow with your palm heel or your forearm. If the assailant is wearing long sleeves, another option is to grab a sleeve and do not let go while simultaneously moving your body into a rearmount. From the rearmount, you can pummel your assailant with your free arm using punches, hammerfists, forearm, blows, and vertical elbow strikes while being sure to control the edged-weapon arm.

Once you have inflicted your initial damage on the assailant, you can stand up to stomp his head preferably on his deadside (away from the edged-weapon arm). Another option from the mount is to reach around with your free arm to grip the assailant's head for a severe neck torque. While using the neck torque takedown, you can also roll back with the assailant to switch positions into a top mount and to turn the edged weapon against the assailant.

Hook Stab or Slash Defense with the Defender on His Back

If the assailant tries a right-hook stab (looping the edged weapon around, similar to a roundhouse punch), use a body defense moving away from the stab (similar to our face-to-face standing defense) turning onto your left hip with a simultaneous counterattack.

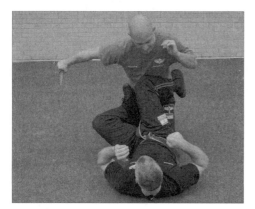

Figure 4.21a

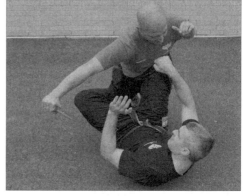

Figure 4.21b

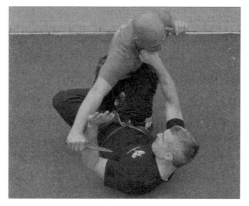

Figure 4.21c

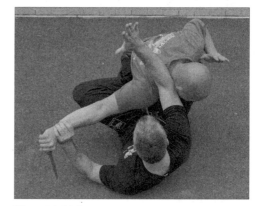

Figure 4.21d

Figures 4.21a–d. Block the attack with your left-arm while moving your body away from the incoming stab while simultaneously counterattacking with your right arm to the attacker's throat, jaw, nose, or eyes.

Another option, if your timing is good, is to bring your nearside knee up to touch your sameside elbow to block the assailant's arm at the elbow while delivering a strike to the throat, jaw, nose, or eyes. While this technique option can present a challenge in controlling the edged-weapon arm, the bottom line is to use whatever technique option works for you to block and secure the edged weapon-wielding arm. Again, most importantly, with any blocking option, immediately assert control over the edged-weapon arm.

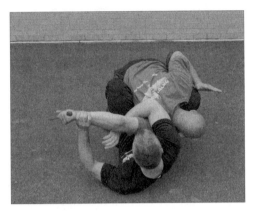

Figure 4.21e

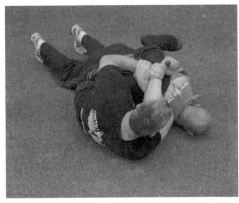

Figure 4.21f

Figures 4.21e–f. Use a modified Control Hold A to control his edged-weapon arm while switching from your left hip to your right hip. Clamp down hard on his shoulder and continue to turn on your side to gain maximum positional control of the weapon, especially if you can establish a closed guard. Another option to avoid pinning your leg underneath the assailant using Control Hold A is to swing your bottomside leg forward as you apply the lock allowing you to place both legs atop the assailant's back for control.

Recall, an alternative defense variation (covered previously in Chapter 3) is to disengage immediately after the block and counterattack by inserting your feet in between you and the assailant for heel kicks to knock him backward, and then quickly transition to your feet. However, if you do not knock the assailant significantly backward, this disengagement without controlling the weapon runs the risk of having your legs stabbed or slashed.

Lower Body Stab with the Defender on His Back
This is a very difficult attack to defend because of the short distance between the edged weapon to your groin and midsection. Using your legs to knock the assailant backward is certainly one preemptive defense. This technique is represented in Figures 4.22a–d.

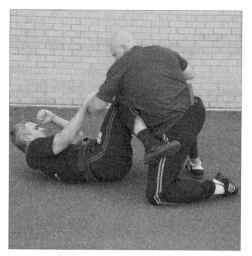

Figure 4.22a

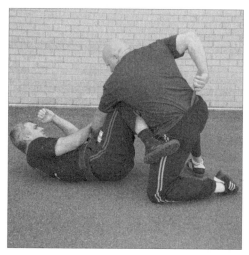

Figure 4.22b

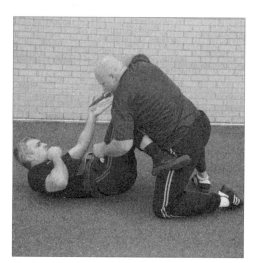

Figure 4.22c

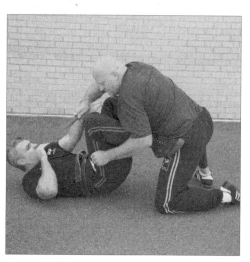

Figure 4.22d

Figures 4.22a–d. Deflect-redirect the edged weapon (similar to our standing defense against an extremely close low stab previously represented in Figures 3.06a–b) with your sameside hand. Using the web of your sameside hand, slap the back of the assailant's handgrip. Parry the edged weapon away while turning your torso onto your hip to aid in the deflection-redirection while creating a body defense.

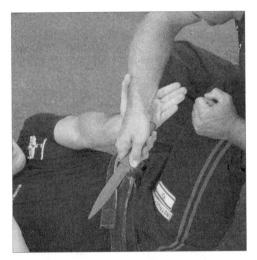

Figure 4.22e

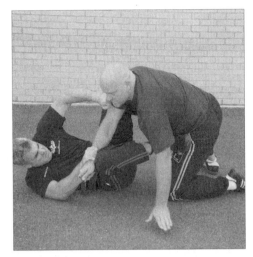

Figure 4.22f

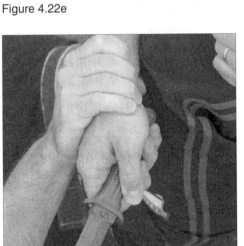

Figure 4.22g

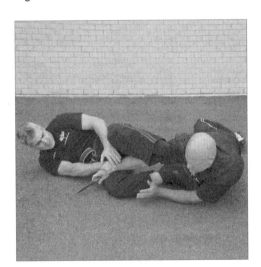

Figure 4.22h

Figures 4.22e–h. Parry the thrust away while using a slight body defense. Immediately try to control or pin the edged-weapon arm with your other arm and your nearside knee by clamping them together as the edged weapon is deflected away from your body. Use your free arm (the arm that initially deflected the edged weapon) and legs to attack the assailant in the head. Be sure to control the weapon if you maintain contact with him.

After the initial defense, a straight armbar to break or dislocate the elbow is an option but, in any event, be sure to control the edged weapon. Note: You could also use the "L" block against this type straight stab to complete the defense, but this particular deflection is quicker. If an attacker tried to stab you in the face while on the ground, the L-block (covered next) is the preferred defense because it provides more of a deflection area. It can be used because you have more time as the weapon must travel a greater distance to reach your head area.

Stab to the Throat with the Defender on His Back

This is another difficult attack to defend because of the short distance between the edged weapon and your throat. Using your legs to knock the assailant backward is a preferred defense.

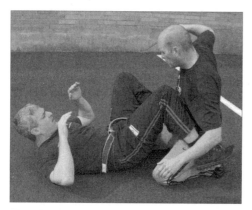

Figure 4.23a

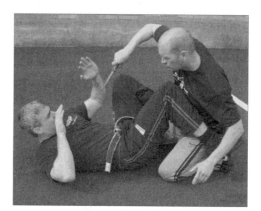

Figure 4.23b

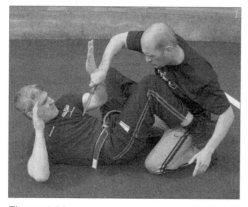

Figure 4.23c

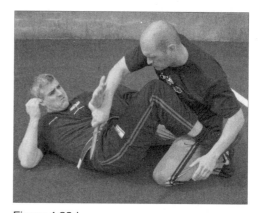

Figure 4.23d

Figures 4.23a–d. Redirect-deflect the edged weapon (similar to the standing "L" block defense against a straight stab previously represented in Figures 4.07a–e) with your deflecting arm bent at an approximately seventy-degree angle. As you parry, move your torso slightly to the left to help create a body defense. The parrying movement leads the body's defensive movement. Once again, the deflection-redirection is no more than a four- to six-inch movement diagonally out. The defensive movement is not an uncontrolled swipe. The defensive arm uses the entire length of the forearm from the pinky to the elbow to deflect any change in the height of the stab attempt. The movement rotates the wrist outward so that your left thumb, kept attached to the hand with all the fingers pointing up, turns away from you as contact is made with the opponent's arm to redirect the incoming thrust. After the parry is made and without breaking contact with the assailant's arm, hook the assailant's arm by cupping your left hand, wrapping your left thumb around his forearm for control and pinning the arm against the assailant's torso while delivering debilitating counterpunches to the throat or jaw.

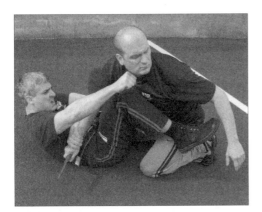

Figure 4.23e

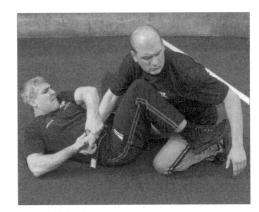

Figure 4.23f

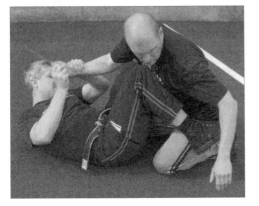

Figure 4.23g

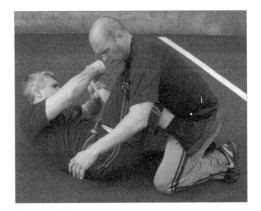

Figure 4.23h

Figures 4.23e–h. Caption continue on next page

Figures 4.23e–h. The objective is to avoid being stabbed while placing you to the assailant's deadside with simultaneous combatives setting up Cavalier #1.

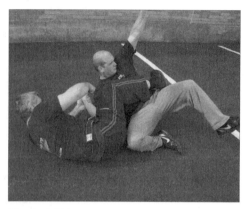

Figure 4.23i

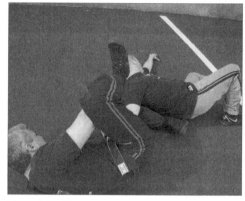

Figure 4.23j

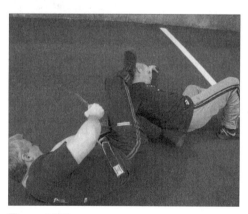

Figure 4.23k

Figures 4.23i–k. Combined Cavalier #1 with a scissors sweep is depicted. To sweep the assailant, drop your left leg to the ground placing your heel against the assailant's lower leg while hooking the assailant's torso with your right leg. Once your legs are in position, kick across your body with your right leg while applying torquing pressure to the assailant's wrist. As you sweep the assailant onto his back, use heel kicks to neutralize the threat while stripping the edged weapon from his grip.

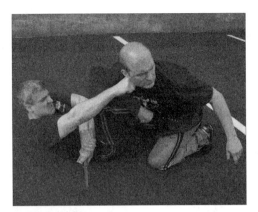

Figure 4.23l

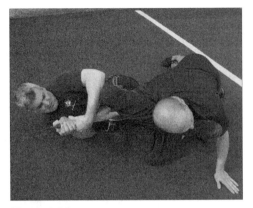

Figure 4.23m

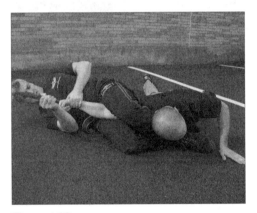

Figure 4.23n

Figures 4.23l–n. You may also apply a straight armbar rather than moving into the sweep technique by swinging your left leg in front of the assailant's face. As you cross-face him with your left leg, trap his weapon arm with your right thigh squeezing both thighs together. Maintain strict control of the weapon keeping the arm pressed against your torso with the blade perpendicular to your torso. Using your core, arch your back to break his arm while simultaneously stripping the edged weapon from his grip.

Defenses Against a Needle

Defending against an attack with a needle uses the same edged-weapons defenses you have now learned, but you must take great care not to be jabbed because of the great risk of contracting an infectious disease.

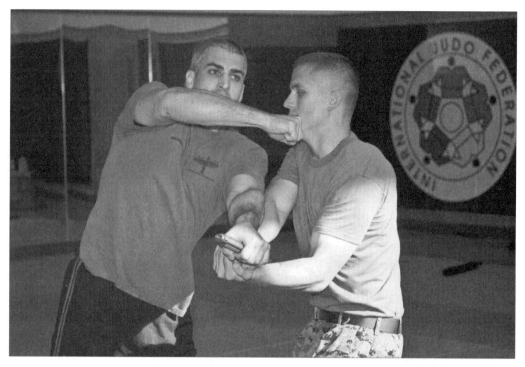

Training U.S. Marines. Photo courtesy of USMC Combat Camera.

CHAPTER 5

Handgun Defenses

If someone pulls a gun on you and does not shoot, he or she wants something. It is possible that he or she *may* still shoot you, but not before achieving a desired ends. When possible, compliance with the gunman's demands is the best solution. Compliance, however, is not always possible; especially, if your instinct tells you the gunman intends you bodily harm no matter what. Carefully consider your options and course of action. Again, there may be situations in which attempting a disarm is impossible and you must comply with the gunman's wishes. Firearms are often referred to in krav maga parlance as "hot weapons."

Similar to our previous edged-weapon defenses described in Chapter 4, to defend a firearm threat you must deflect-redirect the weapon using a body defense and move off the line of fire combined with simultaneous combatives to facilitate the disarm. Krav maga's overriding philosophy is to give you any and every advantage. You might have to wait until the assailant closes the distance or lowers his guard in response to your feigned acquiescence, when, in fact, you are simply waiting for the best opportunity to disarm him. Be aware of your surroundings and how they might affect your disarm including walls, curbs, parked vehicles, the confines of a small space such as an elevator, or a vehicle, and your footing. With all firearms disarms, carefully gauge the distance and your reach capability to deflect-redirect and secure the weapon. When distance allows, krav maga's handgun defenses are readily applicable against tasers, stun-guns and aerosol-type weapons.

If the assailant has a handgun and you decide to run, the greater the distance between you and the gunman, the more likely you will not be hit. Obviously, a bullet moves faster than any human reaction. Handguns are difficult to fire with accuracy at longer ranges and only skilled shooters can fire with accuracy at distance. Fortunately, criminals tend not to be the best shots, but the high-capacity pistol magazines give them up to seventeen chances or more to hit you.

Shooting Accuracy at Close Range

It is helpful to envision several scenarios in which an assailant could deploy a firearm against you—and avoid them in real life. Of course the best defense against a firearm or any type of weapon is to avoid a situation that exposes you to danger. Common sense

151

should always prevail. Going to an ATM at night alone does not make good common sense. Venturing into a parking lot without scanning your environment, or parking in an unlit area or in a non-heavily trafficked area are also not good strategies. You must envision as many negative-five scenarios as possible. Do your best to plan or envision what you might do if faced with these extreme life-threatening circumstances. These scenarios could include a gunman surfacing from behind a neighboring parked car as you begin to enter your vehicle or confronting you from behind as you insert the key into your front door. Most criminals seek the element of surprise and plan accordingly.

> For krav maga founder, Imi Lichtenfeld, a subtle fundamental training tenet emerged: the direct correlation between mental imagery and physical ability. As an example of mental training, think about the following scenarios and how you might react:
>
> 1) You are alone and entering your vehicle in a parking lot with vehicles parked to both sides and the front of your vehicle. An assailant armed with a handgun darts from behind the parked vehicle on your driver side and holds the firearm six inches from your back.
>
> 2) In a similar scenario, the assailant holds the firearm six inches from the back of your head.
>
> 3) The assailant holds the firearm to the side of your head in front of your ear while he is positioned in front of the rear passenger door.
>
> 4) It is late in the evening and the parking lot is deserted. The assailant, armed with what seems to be a handgun, stands three feet behind you and orders you to put your keys on the roof and move away from the vehicle. (This is very likely a strict compliance scenario unless you feel he intends you bodily harm no matter what.)
>
> 5) You are putting a child in the rear seat and an assailant approaches similar to Scenario #1 above.
>
> Continue to develop similar mental training scenarios taking into consideration multiple variables such as confined spaces between vehicles that may limit your movement.

For example, many modern vehicles have remote keys. Perhaps, rather than facing your vehicle as you prepare to enter it, it might be wise to "about face" to make sure no one is attempting to sneak up on you from the rear. You should also check in the backseat of your vehicle before entering it. Assess your surroundings and how a weapon disarm will be affected if your car is parked close to another car limiting the armed opponent's movement along with your movement.

If you flee, run in a non-linear pattern as fast as possible. In other words, flee using a zigzag pattern to make yourself a more difficult target or locate cover to stop a bullet such as a building or the engine block of a vehicle. A gunman has more difficulty swinging his gun-arm and body in the direction of his dominant arm to shoot accurately. If you are facing a right-handed gunman and you decide to turn and run, move laterally to your right—it is more difficult for him to swing the gun across his body as you run away. When encountering a left-handed gunman, as you turn to run, move to your left. These evasions are also applicable for rifle/and submachine guns (SMGs).

Notably, trained law enforcement professionals when under the stress of a violent encounter often achieve less than a twenty percent hit rate according to the FBI. It is the author's opinion that such statistics should not be interpreted as criticism of these departments' professionalism. Rather, these facts underscore the realities of a violent, often surprise encounter. You can therefore extrapolate that if you must run, it is a fair assumption that you may reach safety unscathed.

In an active shooter situation, it is preferable to begin your evasion plan (or a disarming technique) as soon as the threat is recognized. In short, non-telegraphed (body movements indicating what you are going to do before you actually do it) and unpredictable evasive maneuvers improve your chance of successfully disarming him or fleeing respectively.

If you cannot flee the active shooter scene, find cover or concealment. There is a difference between cover and concealment. Cover effectively shields you from incoming fire. Concealment hides you but is not impervious to gunfire. If you are located within reach of the gunman and you conclude fleeing or reasoning with him is futile, you must use the appropriate disarming technique. If you find yourself in an active shooter situation and you cannot close the distance for a disarming technique, you can throw objects at the gunman such as bags, books, chairs, staplers, coins, etc. to either close the distance for a disarm or as distractions in your attempt to flee. If you are hit, you may wish to feign being dead to prevent the shooter from pumping more rounds into you, but under no circumstances should you give up. Remember, many victims die because they lose the will to live.

In an active shooter situation within a crowd, one disarm technique, requiring great nerve, is to upend the shooter. Close on him from behind, reach down and clasp his legs just above ankles and brace one shoulder against his buttocks and yank sharply backward to dump him on his head. The assailant will let go of the weapon or, if he holds onto it, likely break his wrists on impact. As a last resort, a number of the intended victims may swarm the gunman throwing anything they can at him to overwhelm him. This tactic, for untrained people and sometimes trained people alike, is contrary to human nature. Without a determined brave soul to initiate and rally the group into action, this strategy is unlikely to succeed.

Active Shooter

Below are ten common sense suggestions if you find yourself in an active shooter situation. Try not to panic, think clearly, and ...

1) If the gunman is shooting in all directions, find cover—something that will stop high-powered bullets. Drop any objects that weigh you down or hinder your movement.

2) If you cannot find cover, drop immediately to the ground and scan again for cover.

3) If you are behind cover and you feel the need to locate the gunman or gunmen's location(s), do not break your cover at torso height; rather, peek around your cover keeping low to the ground. You may wish to look for an improvised weapon such as rock or something hard to throw at him or hit him if he approaches and you have no other recourse.

4) The two-to-three-second rush rule suggests that fleeing by short running bursts for two to three seconds in a non-linear pattern, and then finding cover, hinders the gunman's properly acquiring you as a target. Try to run in a low crouch but not so low that you cannot maintain speed.

5) If you decide to stay put, do not crouch down; lie down. By crouching, you could be mistaken by responding security personnel as an armed assailant. Do not assume you will be recognized as an innocent.

6) If you have to go around a building corner, do it quickly. If the shooter is there or there is another shooter, your quick appearance should surprise him, and provided the distance is appropriate, you may attempt a disarm or if the distance is greater, find other cover or double back.

7) Windows present dangers. Obviously, glass can be shot through and the bullet(s) may spray shattered glass on you.

8) If you are behind cover and the shooter is targeting you, if you want to see where he is, peer around your cover but exit from a different place. The shooter might naturally expect you to egress from your initial vantage point. Escaping from another location might throw his reaction time and, consequently, his aim off.

9) Secluding yourself in shadows can provide concealment.

10) Do not silhouette yourself. Placing your darker outline between the shooter and a lighter background can attract attention.

Krav Maga's Firearm Disarm Philosophy

The brain slows down when processing several stimuli or engaged in two thought processes. If you must disarm an assailant brandishing a weapon—in this case a firearm—the most opportune time to act is when the assailant is distracted or first deploying the firearm. He or she may be giving you an order or responding to your entreaty not to harm you. You might also spit in the assailant's face or use another distraction such as throwing loose change, keys, or anything else that is handy to initiate the disarm.

Keep in mind, if you do attempt to disarm the assailant, he or she now considers you a deadly threat and will fight as if his or her life is at stake. Firearms are ergonomically designed for the operator—not someone trying to take the weapon away, especially, if the operator has a two-handed vise grip on it. Therefore, whenever possible, you must move deep to the assailant's deadside. In nearly every instance, the firearm will discharge as you deflect-redirect it because of the assailant's reflexive flinch-trigger-pull response. Do not worry about this. Your deflection-redirection hand will not get hurt.

Prioritize securing the weapon while simultaneously debilitating your assailant with combatives to the throat, groin, eyes, and other secondary targets. As always, your krav maga must be decisive and brutally efficient. In addition, you need to secure the firearm in the best possible way reducing the chances of bystanders being shot. Keep in mind that the assailant's immediate instinctive or "flinch" response will be to retract his gun and pull the trigger. Therefore, your strategy must also incorporate "time in motion." Time in motion is the movement pattern where physically the firearm (or any other type of weapon) is likely to end up because of your deflection-redirection and the assailant's reflexive response. Once again, the need to move deep to the deadside is evident to keep yourself clear of the weapon's line of fire.

Basic Firearms Knowledge

It is helpful to have a basic understanding of firearms. There are two types of handguns, revolvers and semi-automatics, with the latter in greater circulation these days. A revolver uses a rotating cylinder to cycle the next round into the chamber while a semi-automatic uses a spring-loaded clip that pushes another round into the chamber as the previous round is ejected. A revolver usually holds 5–8 rounds while a semi-automatic can hold from 8–17 rounds of ammunition. Some high capacity magazines can hold more than 17 rounds. If you disarm a gunman by securing the barrel at the trigger-well and his finger is on the trigger, a semi-automatic handgun is likely to discharge. Krav maga frontal handgun defenses secure the slide preventing the ejection of the spent round rendering the gun temporarily inoperable. In the case of a revolver, securing it at the trigger guard while wrapping the hand around the cylinder can prevent it from cycling a new round as well.

It is best to work with an expert to educate yourself on firearms operations, especially, to learn how to clear the weapon and make it operational. This ability could be crucial after you have disarmed the assailant and created distance described more fully in the upcoming techniques, specifically Figures 5.01. You should learn how to "tap and rack" a handgun to ready it for use or put it "in battery." When a firearm is not operational, it is called "out of battery."

Once you have secured the handgun, the standard krav maga operating procedure is to tap the magazine from the bottom (the insertion point into the grip), and then turn the handgun parallel to the ground to check the ejection port and rack a new round. After redirecting-deflecting and securing a semi-automatic handgun, rotate it ninety degrees, allowing gravity to help dispense a spent cartridge's case that has likely jammed the weapon. Even if you do not tap and rack the handgun, you should still consider the handgun "live" or functional for safety purposes, particularly, if you use it for cold-weapon combatives.

After you create separation from the assailant, you can use the handgun as a tool—but not your only tool—to fend off additional attacks. For example, if the assailant continues aggressive actions toward you, you can straight kick him in the groin, sidekick him in the knee, or use the handgun to strike him in the head always keeping the muzzle pointed toward him. Simply consider the handgun an extension of your body, but do not allow the barrel to face any part of your body. Importantly, if you have your own firearm, you should revert to using it rather than the assailant's for the obvious reasons that you are familiar with it and have confidence in it.

Keep in mind that you might not know if the firearm is real or functional. It could be a starter pistol or "airsoft" type of facsimile weapon. One of the dangers of using an unfamiliar firearm is that it could explode in your hand. Criminals are not always the brightest and a live round could be loaded in a starter pistol. If you rack and tap the weapon while loading a live round into a starter pistol and pulling the trigger, the results could be disastrous for you. One indicator that the weapon is functional is if you immediately order the assailant down to the ground and he or she complies. An opposite indicator suggesting the weapon is inoperative is if the assailant ignores your commands and rushes at you in which case you need to use your krav maga combatives. If you decide to shoot the assailant, shoot center mass. If the assailant is wearing body armor, shoot him in the head or multiple times into the same location of the bulletproof vest. Your first shot will damage the body armor and the successive shots may penetrate the vest.

Note: All of the following techniques assume the handgun is held by the assailant's right arm.

The Four Essential Components of Gun Defenses

Disarming an assailant armed with a firearm can be extremely difficult. Be sure that you have exhausted all compliance options and that you have no choice but to attempt the disarm technique. If you decide there is no choice but to disarm an assailant, you must follow the four pillars of krav maga's firearm defenses:

1) Redirect-deflect the weapon combined with a simultaneous body defense to move you off the line.

2) Control the firearm whenever possible moving deep to the deadside while stunning and neutralizing the assailant.

3) Understand "time in motion"—or what the gunman's reaction will be the instant you react.

4) Disarm the assailant and create distance using the firearm to your best advantage.

There are myriad angles and heights that an assailant could threaten you with a firearm. The following disarm techniques cover the positions and angles handguns are most commonly used by an assailant. These are simply presented as a blueprint against firearm threats. Krav maga's philosophy is to adapt to a situation using core techniques and principles. If you find yourself in a situation not covered in this book, fall back on the four pillars for firearm defenses and use common sense to prevail. Notably, you could find yourself defending against a handgun threat covered or obscured by a magazine, newspaper, or cloth. The defenses remain the same, but take into account that your grip and subsequent control on the handgun could slip from the weapon if the angle of deflection-redirection and control is incorrect. Importantly, if you attempt a disarm, the assailant is likely to instinctively retract his arm. You must understand time in motion—both yours and his—or how a body instinctively reacts to a stimulus to properly time and execute a firearm disarm.

We will examine five different distances throughout the various firearm defenses:

1) The firearm is extended from the assailant's torso and held at a distance but within arm's length of you.

2) The firearm is held close to the assailant's torso but within arm's length of you.

3) The firearm is extended from the assailant's torso and the muzzle is making physical contact with your body.

4) The firearm is held close to the assailant's torso and the muzzle is in physical contact with your body.

5) The firearm is not yet deployed and you are in arm's length of the potential assailant.

Author's Note: Due to pictorial constraints, for certain Chapter 5 techniques, the initial deflections-redirections are depicted; however, the final take away process is omitted because it is the same for all frontal disarms moving to an opponent's deadside. Be sure to thoroughly understand the Figures 5.01 disarm procedure because it will be referenced to finish many techniques.

Note: For all firearm defenses, the gunman is likely to pull the weapon back to thwart your attempted control while pulling the trigger to discharge the weapon.

For demonstration purposes only, the handgun is often held without the trigger finger inserted to prevent injury. Where necessary, the "assailant" has inserted his finger to show the specific removal technique. When practicing these techniques, determine with your partner if he or she will keep the trigger finger inserted.

Handgun Defenses from the Front

Frontal Handgun Defense #1

When an assailant threatens you from the front and if you decide to disarm him, you must gauge the distance between the firearm and your reach to safely control it. It does not matter if the assailant has one or two hands on the handgun grip. Neither does the level of the handgun, provided you can close the distance, deflect-redirect, and secure the firearm. Note though, that if the assailant has the gun in one hand, he could blade his body creating a different angle of counterattack for you. In addition, with a two-handed grip, the assailant can better resist a disarm underscoring the need for deep deadside movement combined with strong debilitating combatives to the head. Also, note that a two-handed grip leaves his head wide open for your counterattacks. If the assailant is within your reach, now consider your timing. If you must react (assuming the gun is in the assailant's right hand), begin with a subtle forward lean.

Just prior to launching your disarm, punch out with your left hand to deflect and secure the barrel just in front of the trigger guard, locking your deflecting-redirecting arm out. Place your full weight on the weapon while simultaneously counterattacking the neck or head. Optimally, control the barrel by keeping it parallel to the ground for maximum control, especially if the assailant attempts to rip it from your grip. You may find depending on both your height and the assailant's height, the barrel may be forced slightly up or slightly down. If you are taller, because of the defense's design, your controlling grip will force the barrel slightly downward. If you are shorter, your grip will likely force the barrel upward.

Deflect and control the handgun close to the trigger guard for two reasons. First, controlling the weapon at the trigger guard provides a strong grasp of the weapon for better control, especially if it has a short barrel. The grasp provides for closer leverage to the handgun's grip. Second, if the handgun is compensated or has holes in the barrel to allow more gas to escape to reduce the recoil, by securing the weapon at the trigger guard your hand will not be burned by the escaping gasses.

The deflection-redirection of the handgun is done by inserting the web of your hand (in between your thumb and index finger) into the front section of the trigger guard. You are punching the handgun away, not slapping it away. This movement will allow your hand to automatically close around the gun deep enough to avoid the muzzle blast (the bullet's exit point on the gun).

Much is written about handgun defenses. One method often suggested is that you should purposefully keep your hands raised indicating compliance. The correct defense simply depends on what position you find yourself—just be sure to keep your elbows close to your sides. Your goal is to create "zero perception" for the assailant beyond your seeming compliance. In other words, you do not want him to have any indication that you intend to disarm him.

Think of the initial deflection-redirection as punching the gun away while holding on to it rather than simply pushing it away. Because the chambered round is likely to fire, you must blade your entire body to remove it from the line of fire as you simultaneously deflect-redirect it from your body. Properly securing the gun and positioning your body to the deadside is crucial. Many Israeli krav maga imitations make the mistake of deflecting-redirecting the gun and attempting to pin the gun in front of the defender. In other words, the defender does not deflect and move deep enough into the assailant's deadside with the defender's full weight on the weapon, especially if the assailant has a two-handed grip. An assailant with a two-handed grip will obviously have more control over the weapon and strength to resist your disarm. Therefore, proper technique must always prevail. Deflect-redirect the barrel with all of your weight to maintain dominant control of the weapon and keep your grip tight to control the barrel.

Krav maga's deflection-redirection method mechanically jams the semi-automatic handgun's slide mechanism preventing a new round from cycling into the chamber or the cylinder of the revolver from rotating. As you deflect and secure the gun, burst forward and sharply jam the gun into the assailant's waist area with the slide of the gun parallel to his body creating an "elbow kiss." A simultaneous salvo of punches or palm-heel strikes to his head accompanies the deflection-redirection. Your forearm and assailant's gun-arm create a "V" by the underside of your forearm pressing against the topside of his forearm, but not directly on top of his arm. Your elbow must be behind his elbow for the elbow kiss.

Once you have deflected and moved deadside, maintain an elbow kiss while delivering combatives. Be sure to keep your weight firmly pressed down on the barrel of the handgun with your elbow locked to control the weapon. Be sure to place his arm with your full bodyweight on the weapon in a controlled position keeping you off the line of fire and reducing his ability resist—which he is sure to do. You must use strong punches with good wrist alignment and pivoting your hips to transfer your weight, and then explode through the punch.

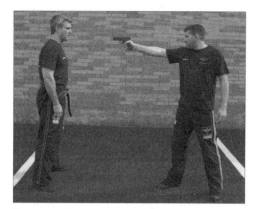

Figure 5.01a

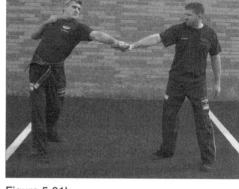

Figure 5.01b

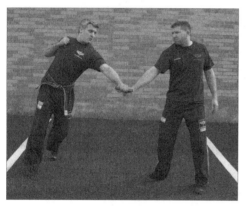

Figure 5.01c

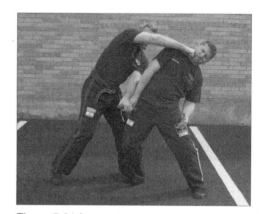

Figure 5.01d

Figures 5.01a–d. Prior to the disarm attempt keep your elbows at your side and try not to look at the weapon. If your elbows are not close to your sides, your impending movement will be more obvious to the gunman. Remain focused on the assailant's face and upper torso. You may slightly shift your weight to the balls of your feet to help propel you forward but not show signs of leaning or swaying forward. If you focus on the weapon, you may telegraph your movements or the assailant might quickly discern your preparation to disarm him and shoot you right away. Only at the instant you launch your disarm, should your eyes laser in on the weapon to deflect-redirect and secure it by locking your arm out for maximum control. This recognition-focus-reaction transition is true of all firearm threats.

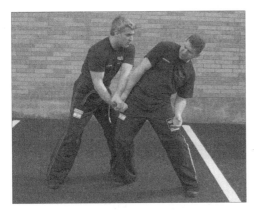

Figure 5.01e

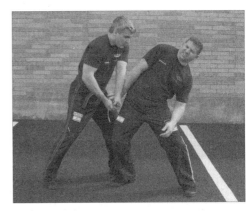

Figure 5.01f

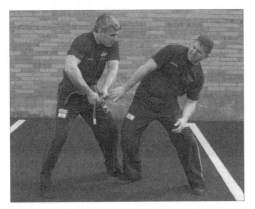

Figure 5.01g

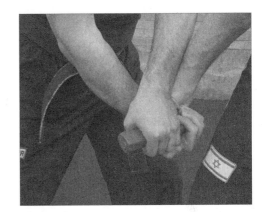

Figure 5.01h

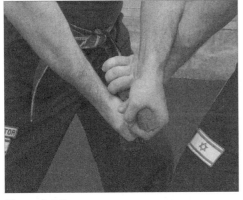

Figure 5.01i

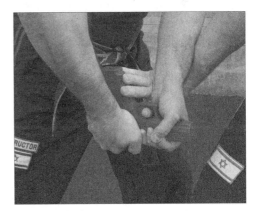

Figure 5.01j

Figures 5.01e–j. Caption on next page

Figures 5.01e–f. Once you have hit the assailant several times (no fewer than three is recommended), maintain your grip on the barrel just above the trigger guard, and then begin the gun takeaway process. Move your other arm close to your nearside hip making sure not to pass any part of you in front of the barrel. With your palm up, secure the rear of the handgun above the grip. Note: On some handgun models there will be an exposed hammer while on others there is no hammer. As you begin to remove the handgun, make sure that both of your hands are gripping the gun strongly for control. With your right hand, rotate/yank the gun back sharply toward your right hip until the handgun grip has rotated a full one-hundred-eighty degrees and is perpendicular to the ground. Pull the handgun back to you by angling the barrel slightly into the assailant to streamline its release from the assailant's trigger finger. This release will likely mangle and break his trigger finger. You may also jolt him with your nearside shoulder while tucking your chin to knock him backward facilitating the release. Immediately create distance between yourself and the assailant because he might now try to disarm you.

While there is a chance that combatives following the firearm deflection-redirection may knock the assailant out, the goal of these strikes is to stun, short-circuit, and unbalance him enough to complete the disarm technique. As with all krav maga techniques, if you do not stun the assailant, he will continue to attack—and you will have an extremely difficult task in disarming him. Remember the gun is ergonomically designed for the assailant to hold, not you. Importantly, if you succeed in your initial deflection-redirection and body defense, as you hit the assailant repeatedly, he is likely to fall or stumble backward pulling the handgun with him. If you are not properly positioned deep to the deadside, the assailant will yank the handgun back and you will still be in the line of fire. In addition, with improper positioning, if your combatives knock the assailant to the ground, you are also in the line of his kicks as he is falling and while he is on the ground. Even if you have jammed the slide, you must not put yourself in the line of fire. Do not make the mistake of redirecting and counterattacking without properly positioning yourself to the assailant's deadside.

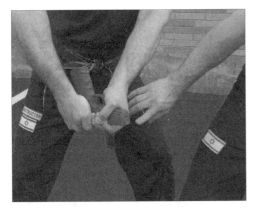

Figure 5.01k

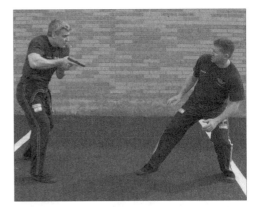

Figure 5.01l

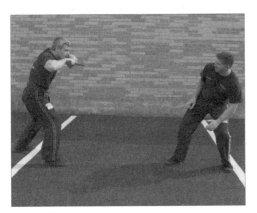

Figure 5.01m

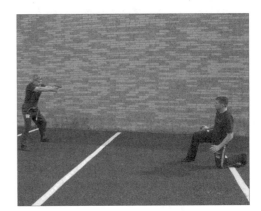

Figure 5.01n

Figures 5.01k–n. If you intend to hold him at gunpoint, as you create proper distance, slap the magazine bottom with the heel of your palm and rack a new round into the chamber or simply run away. In either event, consider how onlookers and, more importantly, law enforcement authorities will view you when running with or brandishing a firearm. You should call the appropriate law enforcement authorities, describe yourself and what you are wearing, and set the firearm down on the ground with your hands clearly visible when they arrive.

Note: This defense can be utilized at three frontal threat heights: midsection, chest, and head. Be aware of variations and the necessary modifications of defending against a small-framed handgun.

Note: For law enforcement personnel, as common sense dictates, you should rely on your own service weapon rather than the assailant's weapon.

If You Miss in Your Initial Attempt to Disarm the Assailant

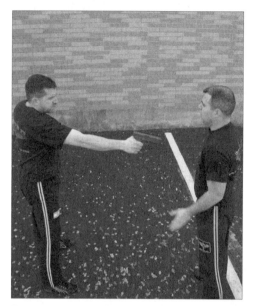

Figure 5.01o

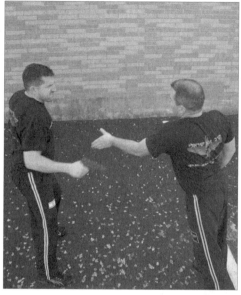

Figure 5.01p

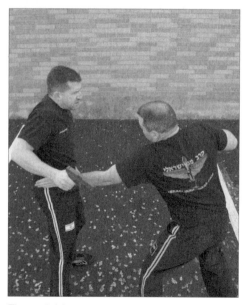

Figure 5.01q

Figures 5.01o–q. If you miss in your initial deflection-redirection or the assailant counters your disarm by retracting or moving the weapon, you must continue to press your defense to acquire control over the handgun. Chances are the assailant will either pull the handgun back directly or circle it to the outside, away from your grasp if he perceives your intent or attempt.

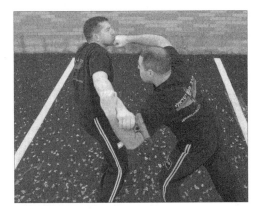

Figure 5.01r

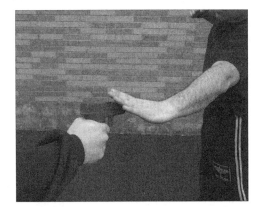

Figure 5.01s

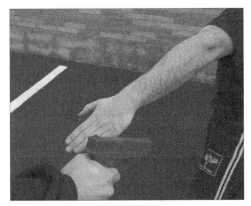

Figure 5.01t

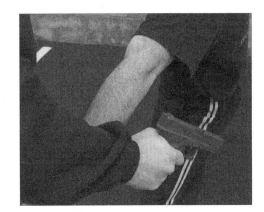

Figure 5.01u

Figures 5.01r–u. If the assailant attempts either one of these counters, continue to close the distance while using the same arm you attempted to disarm him to snake around his gun-arm. Continue combatives with knee counterattacks to the attacker's groin. Remember that a knee strike to the groin will lurch the assailant's body forward. You should use your free arm to brace his neck to prevent his inadvertently head-butting you. Never break contact with the assailant's gun-arm. Always and immediately, secure the arm as close as possible to the gun holder's wrist to prevent the barrel from turning into you or being yanked back—which will be the attacker's instinctive response. The barrel will turn upward toward the sky. Unlike the previous frontal defenses, you are not securing the gun by the barrel. Therefore, the handgun will remain functional until your remove it or it runs out of ammunition.

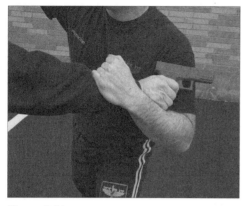

Figure 5.01v

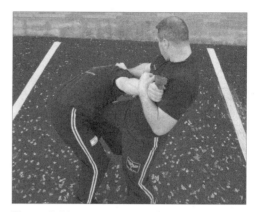

Figure 5.01w

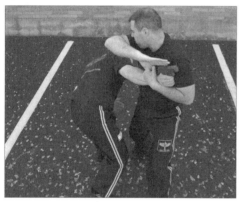

Figure 5.01x

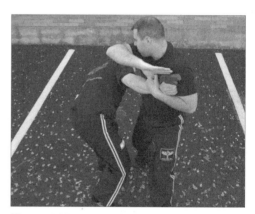

Figure 5.01y

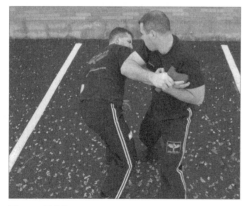

Figure 5.01z

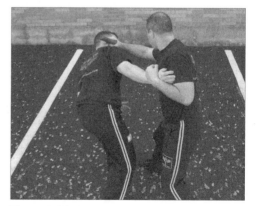

Figure 5.01zz

Figures 5.01v–zz. Once you have secured the gun-arm tightly with your arm wrapped as close to the assailant's wrist as possible, continue with your combatives until you neutralize the threat. After you have debilitated the opponent, maintain a strong vise grip on the assailant's gun-arm, and take your free arm and cross it in front of your face reaching for the handgun's barrel. You should end up with your pinky toward the handgun's sight. Grasp the gun strongly and turn it sharply about ninety degrees with the grip perpendicular to the ground to break the assailant's grip. The barrel should now be perpendicular to the gunman's hand. Once the grip is released, the trigger finger will still be in the handgun's trigger-well. Wrench the gun out and away, which will likely break his trigger finger. You may then use the barrel of the gun to strike the opponent in the head. Again, note if you hit him in the temple, you risk killing him, so use only the force necessary to survive the situation.

Frontal Handgun Defense #1 Modification When the Assailant Falls Backward

This is a modified defense of Frontal Defense #1, when the assailant falls backward as a result of your strong combatives but he still maintains control of the handgun.

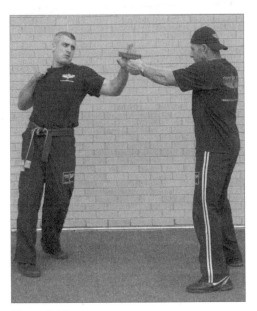

Figure 5.02a

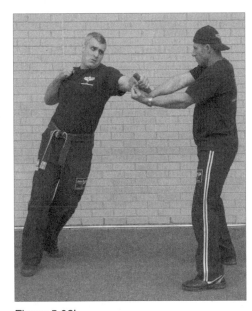

Figure 5.02b

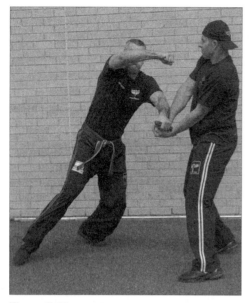

Figure 5.02c

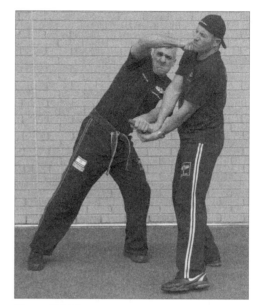

Figure 5.02d

Figures 5.02a–d. During the course of your Frontal Defense #1, you might knock the assailant down but he still might manage to maintain his grip on the weapon, especially if he is gripping the weapon with two hands. This continuum of Frontal Defense #1 reinforces the need to move deadside with a body defense and create a proper elbow kiss. If the defense is not executed correctly, your torso will incorrectly remain in front of the assailant rather than to his deadside. There is a chance you might knock him down and your grip on the barrel could inadvertently release. Notwithstanding the possible jam of the slide as discussed, this puts you squarely in his sights again. Instead, continue to move with him as he falls while maintaining strict control of the handgun. There are a few options to remove the handgun when the assailant is down and is lying on his back.

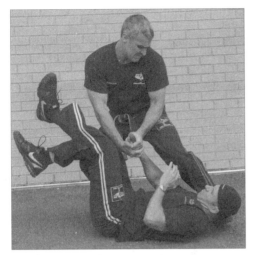

Figure 5.02e

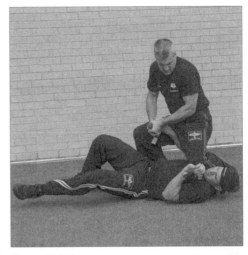

Figure 5.02f

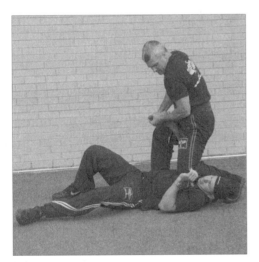

Figure 5.02g

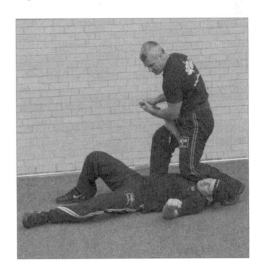

Figure 5.02h

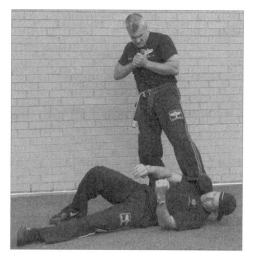

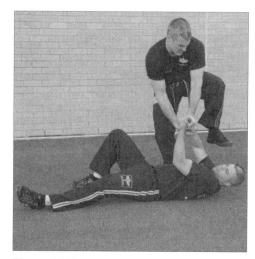

Figure 5.02i

Figure 5.02j

Figures 5.02e–j. To take away the handgun, do not change the grip of your secured left hand. Simply take your right hand and grasp the rear of the slide underneath your left hand as depicted in Figures 5.01h–k. Your right inner palm should fold over your left hand. To remove the weapon from his grip, use your hips and core strength to wrench the handgun's barrel away from you and toward the assailant's torso. After ripping the weapon away from his grip, pull up slightly to disengage it from his mangled trigger finger. Try not to look at the weapon and keep focused on the assailant. Note: You may also use the same takeaway procedure as used in Frontal Defense #1. Another option while maintaining strong control of the barrel is to drop your left knee on the assailant's head and the other knee against his ribs or liver. With both options, your two-handed control of the pistol (regardless of whether the assailant has a one or two-handed grip) affords you great leverage to pry the pistol away. A last option, depicted in Figure 5.02j, is to remain upright and apply two-handed control of the weapon while you stomp on his head with your left heel or drop your left knee and full bodyweight on his head or throat to then remove the weapon.

Frontal Handgun Defense #2

This defense redirects the gun and simultaneously removes the firearm from the assailant's grip. The defender may use frontal Defense #2 if Defense #1 would redirect the line of fire toward a bystander or simply to counter the combined strength of a two-handed handgun grip.

The handgun is once again in the assailant's right hand or could be in both hands. Note again, it does not matter if the assailant has one or two hands grasping the handgun. This defense redirects the firearm in the opposite direction that you learned with Frontal Defense #1. This defense might be used for two reasons: (1) You may simply feel more comfortable with it, or (2) you might be with a companion who would be in the line of fire of Frontal Defense #1's redirection. This double-handed disarm is very powerful and focuses on the weakest part of the assailant's grip: the inner palm rather than against his combined finger clutch strength.

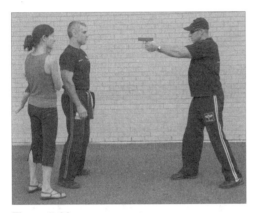

Figure 5.03a

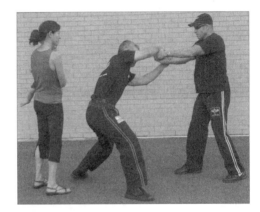

Figure 5.03b

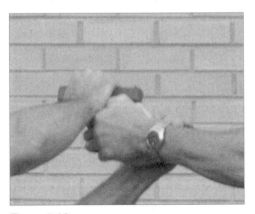

Figure 5.03c

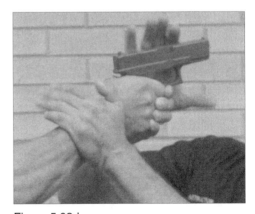

Figure 5.03d

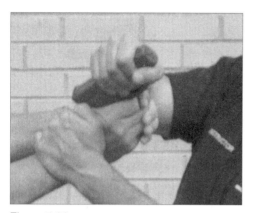

Figure 5.03e

Figures 5.03a–e. There are a few similarities between Frontal Defenses #1 and #2. As with Frontal Defense #1, when an assailant threatens you from the front, if you must disarm him, gauge the distance between the firearm and your reach. If the assailant is within your reach, now consider your timing. Using a subtle forward lean, punch out with your right hand to deflect and secure the handgun by the barrel (the handgun is in the assailant's right hand) while blading your body and simultaneously securing and yanking down sharply on the assailant's gun-arm wrist with your left hand. Keep your left thumb attached to the hand in a "cupping motion." Forcibly punch the handgun through and away from the assailant's grip jarring his gun-arm wrist down to remove the handgun. Be sure to use a simultaneous body defense to move you off the line of fire. Note that Figure 5.03f depicts the technique against a handgun with a flashlight showing how krav maga evolves to counter modern weaponry.

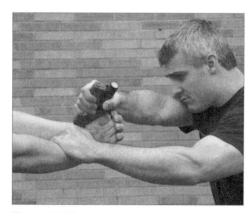

Figure 5.03f

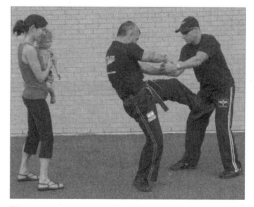

Figure 5.03g

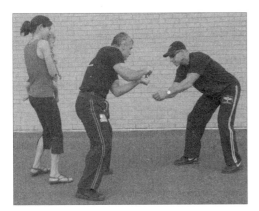

Figure 5.03h

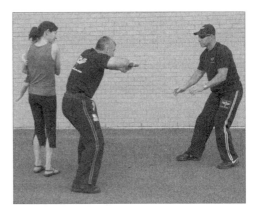

Figure 5.03i

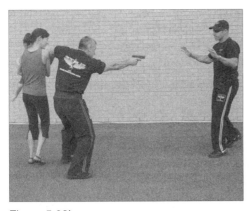

Figure 5.03j

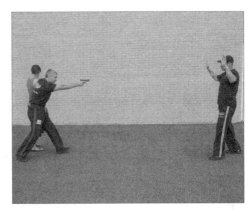

Figure 5.03k

Figures 5.03f–k. Use a near-simultaneous straight kick to his groin with your left leg; then create distance and make the handgun operable. You also have the option of cold weapon combatives to strike the assailant with the barrel in the head or throat immediately after you confiscate it from his grip.

If for some reason you do not succeed at punching the handgun out of his hand(s), relentlessly press the counterattack making sure to stay out of the line of fire. The assailant will likely retract the handgun to pull it away from you. Keep your hands firmly in place and move with his pullback while executing lower body combatives including knees and straight kicks while moving to the assailant's deadside. Do not under any circumstances let go of the handgun. Be careful that the assailant does not hit you with an inadvertent head-butt as a result of your lower body combatives forcing him to lurch forward. Continue your lower body combatives while maintaining strong control of the handgun.

If you have successfully moved to the assailant's deadside while controlling the handgun, you may release your left hand for combatives. One release option is to use a cavalier to keep redirecting the handgun away while exerting great pressure against the assailant's grip. Another option is to control the barrel with your initial deflection-redirection and to release the assailant's wrist to then employ a modified takeaway using the same principles as found in "Frontal Handgun Defense #1." With the barrel firmly secured with your right hand, using an underhand grip, secure the rear of the slide (the only part of the gun that is in between your hand and the assailant's hand) with your left hand. Wrap your fingers around the rear corner of the handgun and yank the rear corner toward you. This will likely break his trigger finger, which, as noted, can be an impediment to your clean release of the handgun from his grip. You must then pull the gun slightly out and away to disengage his mangled finger.

Frontal Handgun Defense Against Handgun on the Assailant's Hip, Under His Garment, or in His Coat Pocket

On the Hip: This defense is similar to Frontal Defense #1; however, the handgun must be controlled and pinned to the assailant's hip. (There is minimal redirection because the assailant's hip impedes the handgun's redirection.)

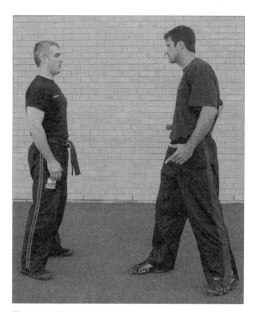
Figure 5.04a

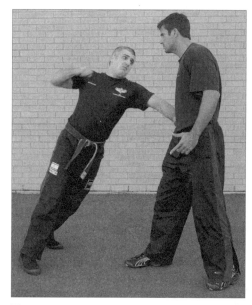
Figure 5.04b

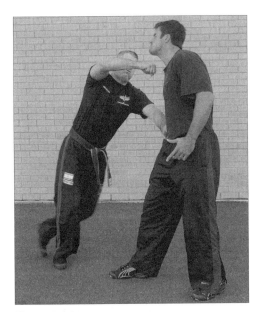

Figure 5.04c

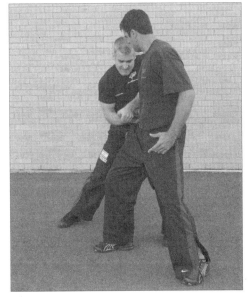

Figure 5.04d

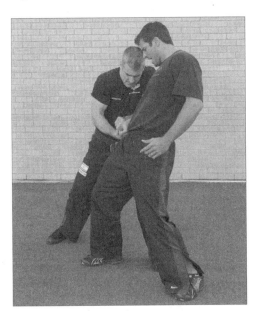

Figure 5.04e

Figures 5.04a–e. This defense uses a simultaneous body defense and control of the handgun with a counterattack to the assailant's head with your free arm. Because the handgun is anchored to the hip, moving to the deadside is once again crucial. As with all weapons defenses, the hand leads the body. The deflection-redirection of the handgun is made using the web of your hand (in between your thumb and index finger) punching it into the front section of the trigger guard while counterattacking with your free arm. This movement will allow your hand to automatically close around the barrel deep enough to avoid the muzzle blast. Think of the initial deflection-redirection as pinning the handgun to the assailant's hip rather than simply pushing it way. Again, properly securing the handgun and positioning your body deadside is critical.

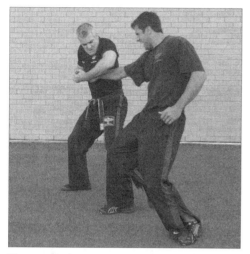

Figure 5.04f

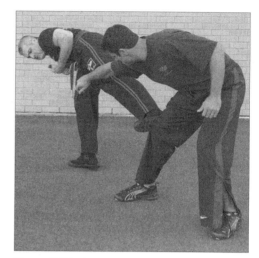

Figure 5.04g

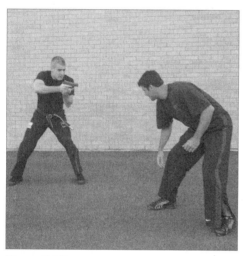

Figure 5.04h

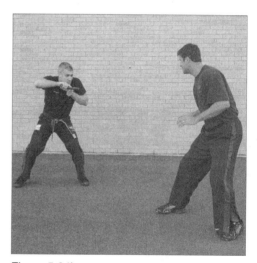

Figure 5.04i

Figures 5.04f–i. To take away the handgun, continue to exert strong control over the barrel. Remove the weapon using the same techniques as learned in Frontal Defense #1 in Figures 5.01.

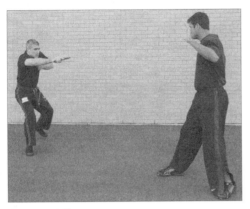
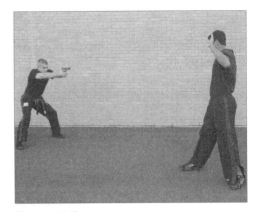

Figure 5.04j

Figure 5.04k

Figures 5.04j–k. Secure the weapon, tap, and rack the weapon to put it back into battery and create distance.

In a Coat Pocket: This defense is similar to the previous defense incorporating elements of Frontal Defense #1, except the handgun's removal differs because you remove the weapon from inside the pocket of an assailant's clothing.

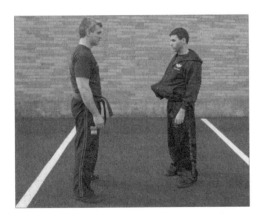
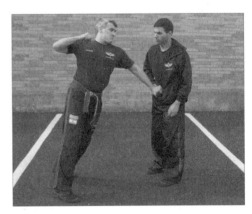

Figure 5.05a

Figure 5.05b

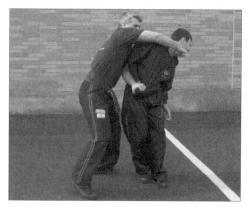

Figure 5.05c

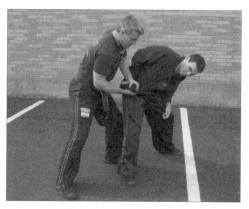

Figure 5.05d

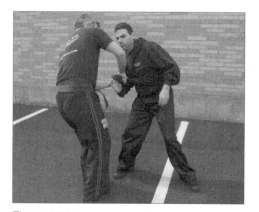

Figure 5.05e

Figures 5.05a–e. Defend this threat similar to your Frontal Defense #1. However, because of the handgun's placement in the pocket, deflect and secure the barrel through the pocket, and then remove it. The firearm is likely to discharge. Again, be aware that the cloth or material can make your hand slide on the barrel and, hence, the importance of moving deadside. If you lose control over the barrel, do not break contact with the handgun. Pin it to the assailant's torso and continue with your combatives. If necessary, use two hands to secure the barrel—clear of the muzzle— while using lower body combatives keeping the barrel pointing away from your legs. After disorienting the assailant with combatives and assuming you still have control of the handgun, keep the barrel pointed away from you, preferably at the assailant. Remove the handgun as learned in Frontal Defense #1 modifying the takeaway to account for the cloth of the pocket.

Under a Garment: This defense is similar to Frontal Defense #1, except the handgun's removal differs because you must remove the weapon from underneath the assailant's clothing.

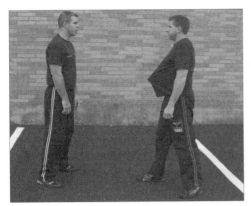

Figure 5.05f

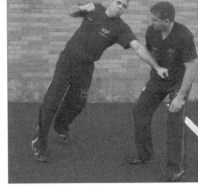

Figure 5.05g

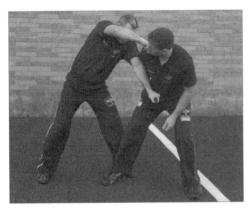

Figure 5.05h

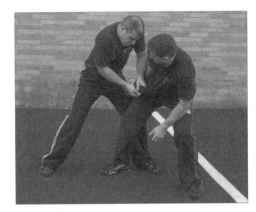

Figure 5.05i

Figures 5.05f–i. Defend this threat similar to your Frontal Defense #1. However, because a garment covers the handgun, you must deflect-redirect and secure the barrel through the garment. Be aware that the cloth or material can make your hand slide on the barrel and, hence, once again, the overriding importance of moving deadside. If you cannot control or lose control over the barrel, do not break contact with the handgun. Pin it to the assailant's torso and continue with your combatives. After disorienting the assailant with combatives and assuming you still have control of the handgun, with your free hand reach under the garment and secure the weapon as directed in Frontal Defense #1. Because you have secured the barrel by grasping the garment, yank down and away on the handgun's hammer portion. Only when you succeed in prying the handgun loose, do you remove your hand from the barrel to quickly then remove the weapon and create distance. Again, you have the option to jolt him with your nearside shoulder while tucking your chin to knock him backward and facilitate the release.

If the assailant tried to bluff you with an extended pointer finger under his garment rather than a real handgun, proceed with the defense while rearranging his finger in the process. Note that a handgun concealed under a newspaper or magazine would be defended similarly, but you must account for slippage of the paper as you secure the barrel.

Frontal Handgun Defense When on Your Knees

If a gunman wants to force you to your knees in "an execution position," it is best to react before you go to your knees. If you are on your knees, use your seeming acquiescence and forward lean to generate momentum into your preferred frontal disarm.

The defense against this threat is similar to Defenses #1 and #2 depending on your preference. I recommend Frontal Handgun Defense #2 which, in turn, offers you two options: to disarm the assailant while on your knees or burst up from your knees into him. Deflect and control the gun while rising on one knee to then burst into the assailant with combatives. For Frontal Defense #1, explode into the assailant keeping control of the weapon to his deadside and continue as you learned in Figures 5.01.

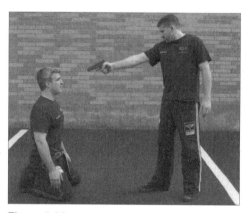

Figure 5.06a

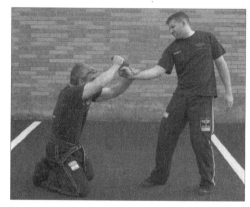

Figure 5.06b

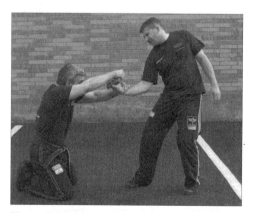

Figure 5.06c

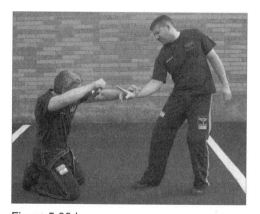

Figure 5.06d

Figures 5.06a–d. For Frontal Defense #2, be sure to move your head off the line of fire. Move your knees as you move off the line of fire while punching the handgun away toward the assailant.

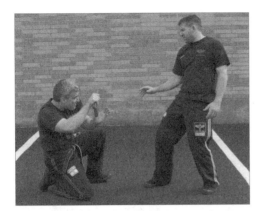

Figure 5.06e

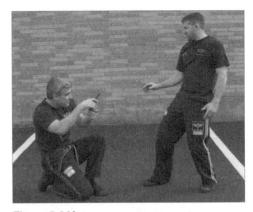

Figure 5.06f

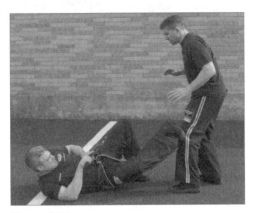

Figure 5.06g

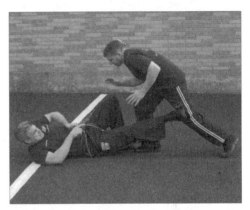

Figure 5.06h

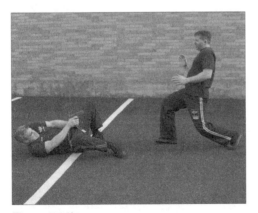

Figure 5.06i

Figures 5.06e–i. Snatch the weapon and fall onto your back while simultaneously tapping and racking the weapon. If necessary, use one leg to ward off the assailant if he rushes at you.

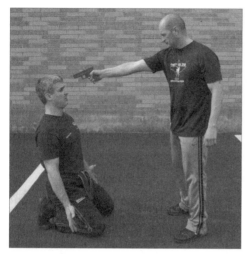

Figure 5.06j

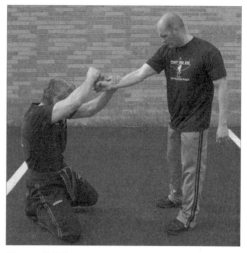

Figure 5.06k

Figures 5.06j–l. As an option, you can kick him in the groin with your left leg and fall onto your back while simultaneously tapping and racking the weapon.

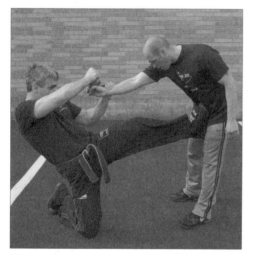

Figure 5.06l

If you botch your initial #1 or #2 defense, and if the assailant pulls the handgun away, as in the standing defenses, determinedly press the defense rising immediately to your feet and close the distance. Continue to burst forward into the assailant, snaking your sameside arm around his gun-arm to secure it while delivering simultaneous combatives including punches, elbows, and knees. Once you have wrapped and secured the gun-arm tightly with your arm snaked as close as possible to the assailant's wrist, continue with your combatives until you neutralize the assailant as depicted in Figures 5.01n–zz.

Frontal Handgun Defense When Shoved Backward

An assailant may become aggressive while holding you at gunpoint and shove you backward using either his free arm or the barrel itself.

Push with His Free Arm: If timed properly, you can use the assailant's push to your advantage. As the assailant pushes, initiate your deflection-redirection and body defense. The defense against this type of assault incorporates elements of Frontal Defense #1 using timing and a bladed body defense to redirect and secure the handgun while taking the assailant out.

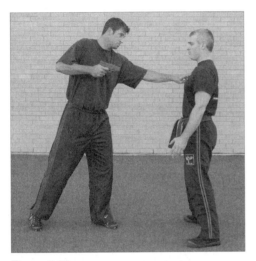

Figure 5.07a

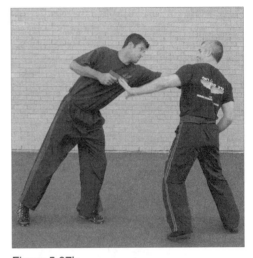

Figure 5.07b

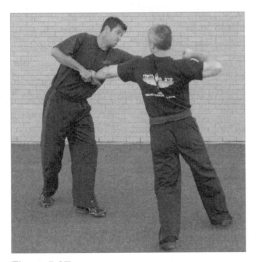

Figure 5.07c

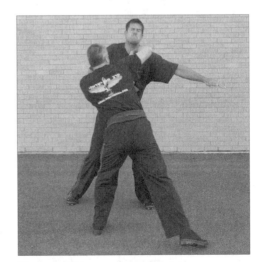

Figure 5.07d

Figures 5.07a–d. Caption on next page

Figures 5.07a–d. By blading your body, the assailant's push with his free arm will miss your torso while you simultaneously deflect-redirect and control the handgun using combatives with your other arm. The deflection-redirection and control of the gun-arm with the simultaneous counterattack is the same as Frontal Defense #1. Blade your body if the assailant tries to push with his free arm. This movement not only defends the push, but also puts you in a superior position to deflect and follow through with Frontal Defense #1. Note: This bladed body defense could also be used against someone pushing you with one or two hands or to avoid colliding with another pedestrian on the street. If the assailant pushes you with the barrel, you may use Frontal Defenses #1 or #2. You may also need to delay your reaction to time it against a second or third push.

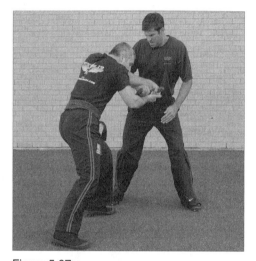

Figure 5.07e

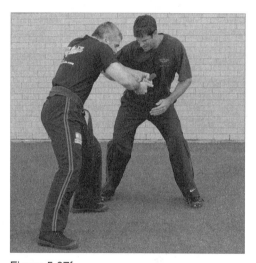

Figure 5.07f

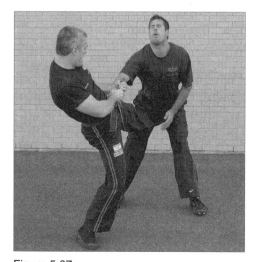

Figure 5.07g

Figures 5.07e–g. Remove the handgun in Frontal Defense #1.

Push with the Barrel: The assailant could also push you with the barrel of the pistol. Use a body defense and simultaneous deflection-redirection of the barrel to assert dominant control and complete the disarm technique.

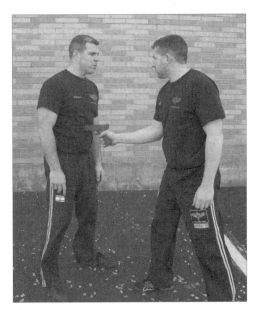

Figure 5.07h

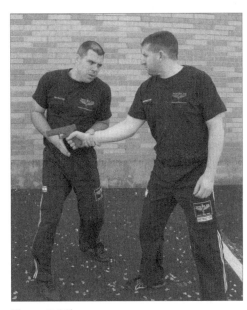

Figure 5.07i

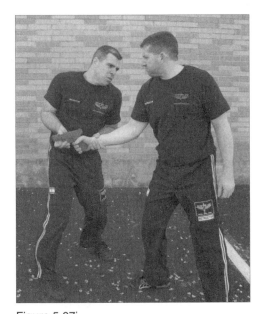

Figure 5.07j

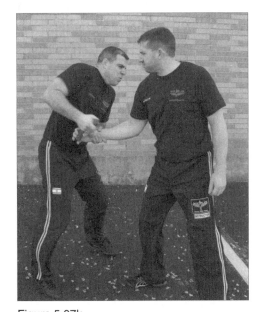

Figure 5.07k

Figures 5.07h–l. Caption on next page

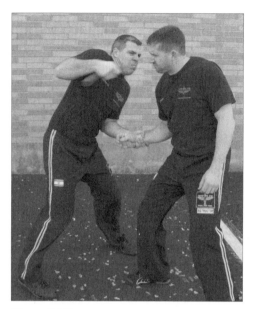

Figure 5.07l

Figures 5.07h–l. As you are forced backward and naturally step to balance yourself, simultaneously bring both arms up to your midsection with palms out and fingertips toward the ground. Your near arm will deflect the assailant's gun-arm away from you by deflecting-redirecting the assailant's wrist while your other far arm is used to clasp the barrel and punch the gun away and out of his hands. Keeping both hands close to your midsection, pivot on the ball of your right foot toward the assailant to exert maximum disarming force, and then immediately strike him in the face, solar plexus, or liver with the barrel.

Another disarm option is to use a simultaneous knee strike to the groin while again making sure to redirect the barrel safely into his midsection. Be sure to keep your torso and hand clear of the line of fire. You may also simply punch the barrel into the assailant's midsection. Use the disarm's powerful momentum to strike the assailant in the midsection with the barrel, preferably, to the liver. On hard contact with his torso, elevate the barrel and use it for a modified uppercut strike to his jaw or throat followed by additional counterattacks.

Frontal Handgun Defense with the Assailant's Other Arm Extended in Front and the Handgun is Pressed to His Hip

An assailant may try to keep you at arm's length with his free arm while threatening you with a handgun placed against his torso at the hip. Note: This is a form of weapon retention that must be considered carefully before acting.

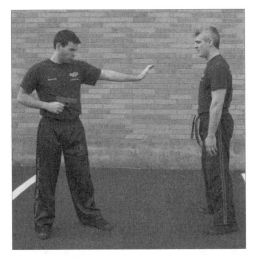

Figure 5.07m

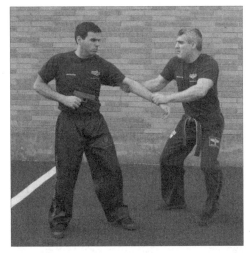

Figure 5.07n

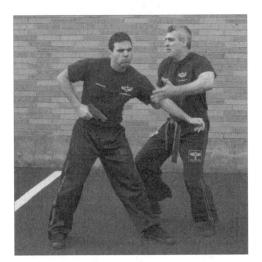

Figure 5.07o

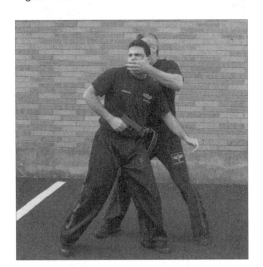

Figure 5.07p

Figures 5.07m–p. This scenario compounds the danger of a handgun disarm because the assailant can use the other arm to ward off your disarm attempt. Nevertheless, if you must react, you can yank the assailant's outstretched arm while simultaneously moving to his deadside to control his head or proceed with a bucket scoop takedown featured in Figures 5.18. If you are not physically overmatched, avoiding going to the ground through the bucket scoop takedown with the assailant is probably the better option.

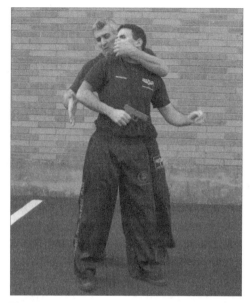

Figure 5.07q

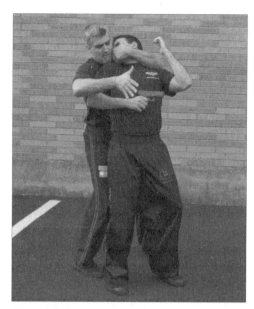

Figure 5.07r

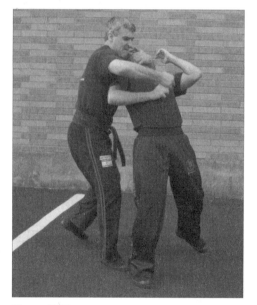

Figure 5.07s

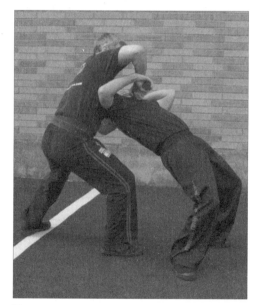

Figure 5.07t

Figures 5.07q–t. By moving behind him, you buy a precious second of time to execute head control with knee combatives to his thighs or a bucket scoop while pinning the firearm to his body. While clearing the line of fire, continue to move behind the assailant while controlling his head to account for the assailant's gun-arm. Secure the handgun at the trigger-well.

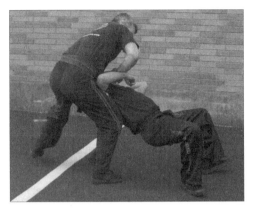

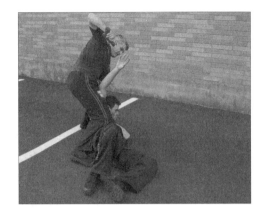

Figure 5.07u   Figure 5.07v

Figures 5.07u–v. Use a modified Cavalier #1 combined with torquing the neck to take him down and punch the handgun out and away from the assailant's grip. You could also use a bucket scoop takedown (covered in Figures 5.18).

Frontal Handgun Defense When Held to the Throat

There are two common situations: first, the handgun is held to throat with the assailant's thumb up with the barrel pointed up to the side of your throat, or, second, the firearm is placed directly under your jaw with the assailant's palm down and the barrel close to your throat. In either case, the assailant might also grab you with his other arm.

The defense against the handgun with the assailant's thumb up is similar to a krav maga choke defense or the defense against an edged weapon held to the side of your neck (see Figures 4.16). As with the edged-weapon threat, the handgun must be controlled carefully using two variations. Your preferred defense variation will depend on two factors: (1) if the opponent is holding you with his free arm, and (2) if you prefer lower body or upper body combatives.

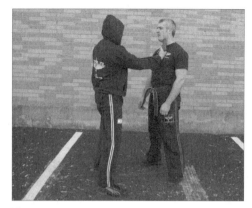

Figure 5.08a

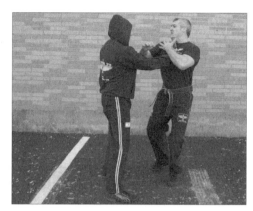

Figure 5.08b

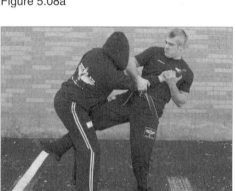

Figure 5.08c

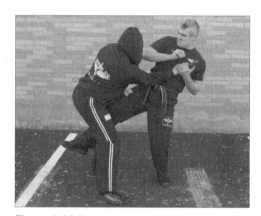

Figure 5.08d

Figures 5.08a–d. For Variation #1, quickly move your head back and away while simultaneously yanking down on the assailant's hand just below the trigger-well on the assailant's four digits to exert great pressure on the wrist forcing the barrel away. While you clear the threat with your nearside arm, your other arm clamps down just above the elbow to further clear you from the barrel and exerts maximum control while simultaneously kicking or kneeing the gunman in the groin. Be sure to exert the modified cavalier correctly to control the handgun with the barrel pointed away from your head. If the assailant uses both arms to grab, you may still use multiple lower body combatives to the groin.

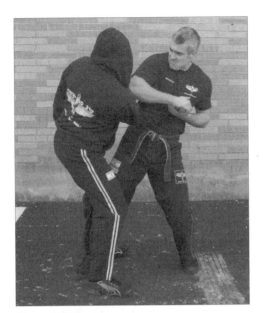

Figure 5.08e

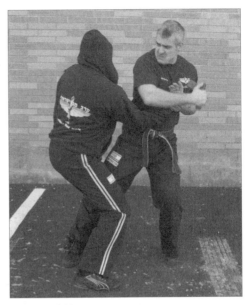

Figure 5.08f

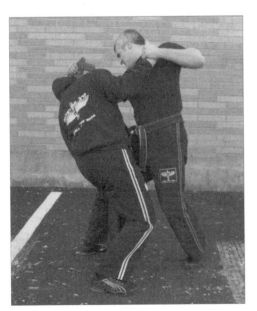

Figure 5.08g

Figures 5.08e–g. The handgun removal is similar to that which you have already learned in Figures 5.01v–zz. Slide your hand across your chest to reach the barrel to dislodge the handgun with a strong grip, prying it down and out to use it as a cold weapon.

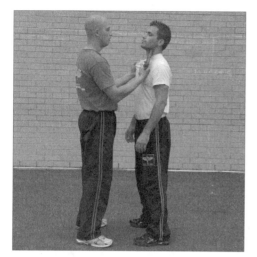

Figure 5.08h

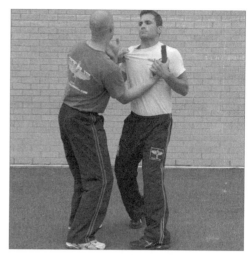

Figure 5.08i

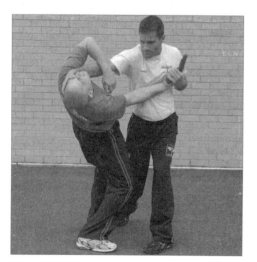

Figure 5.08j

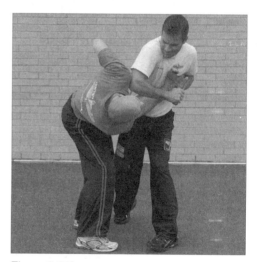

Figure 5.08k

Figures 5.08h–k. If the assailant is holding you with his free arm, for Variation #2, use a body defense to move your head out of the line of fire and using a similar plucking motion to the first defense while embedding your thumb into his eye. Again, the handgun removal is similar to that which you have already learned in Figures 5.01w–zz, except slide your hand across your chest to reach the barrel to dislodge the handgun with a strong grip, prying it down and out to use it as a cold weapon. Note: If you hit him in the temple, you risk killing him, so use only the force you feel necessary to survive the situation.

If the assailant points the gun under your throat with the trigger finger facing you, the defense is similar to Frontal Defense #1 against a threat to the front. Clear your head from the line of fire using a simultaneous barrel deflection-redirection and body defense to remove the threat and secure the weapon. The handgun's removal is the same as Frontal Defense #1.

Frontal Handgun Defenses While on the Ground

When on Your Back

You may be on the ground and on your back while engaged by an assailant who deploys a handgun. Again, the best defense is to prevent the assailant from successfully retrieving the weapon by disabling him with a strike or by using joint locks. As with standing defenses, you need to close the distance, deflect-redirect, and seize control of the weapon. Krav maga's guiding principle is to control the weapon. Recognition and reaction is the key to defeating an edged weapon or firearm in a groundfight.

This is a particularly dangerous situation because the handgun can be deployed and used very quickly, especially amidst a struggle where the assailant is raining down blows on you to distract or disorient you, and then immediately retrieves the handgun. The handgun will usually be secreted in the front or rear of his waistband. It is also possible that he will have a handgun hidden in an ankle holster. Most importantly, if assailant successfully deploys the handgun, no matter which technique you use, it is paramount that you deflect-redirect the line of fire and seize control of the barrel.

If the handgun is hidden in his waistband to the rear, one defensive option is to close the distance and secure his reach arm with Control Hold A, a police hold also often known as a "kimura" hold. To finish the hold and maintain control of the weapon, you need to transition from controlling his forearm to controlling his wrist, and turn the opponent on his side to prevent him from using his free arm to retrieve the weapon as depicted in Figures 4.21e–f. This technique sets up a prone variation of Control Hold A by securing his arm while clamping down on his shoulder and releasing the closed guard momentarily to turn on your side to gain maximum positional control by re-closing the guard. You may also swing your underneath leg atop him to avoid being pinned and use both legs to control him from the top.

Control Hold A places compliance pressure on the opponent's wrist and shoulder. If facing your opponent, or to the side of your opponent, you must secure his right wrist with your left hand. Another option is to grip the flat of the back of his hand by turning your wrist up to create pressure on his wrist keeping the barrel redirected away from you. Raise your wrist up placing upward pressure so that his arm comes up with a ninety-degree bend with fingers toward the ground. Reach over the top of his targeted shoulder, clamping down hard on the shoulder while snaking your right arm over the top of his right arm across his shoulder. Immediately, clasp your other arm. You must clamp down on the shoulder to facilitate the lock. Reach around the arm and encircle it to grip your own forearm. Bring his elbow and wrist close to your body keeping hard pressure on the shoulder by cranking the elbow up and away (to the 2:00 position on a traditional clock) while still keeping it flush against your torso. If he has released the handgun, use your nearside leg to continue exerting pressure on his elbow and release your farside arm to remove the handgun by securing the barrel and wrenching it away similar to the release learned in the handgun defense from the rear.

If the handgun is visible in the front of his waistband and he reaches for it, secure his reaching arm by the wrist to prevent him from deploying the weapon while battering him with your other arm. As with our standing techniques, close the distance to secure the weapon. If he succeeds in partly or completely removing the handgun, you must secure it by the slide.

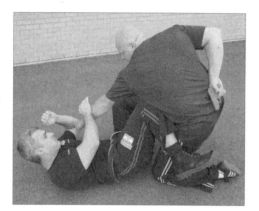

Figure 5.09a

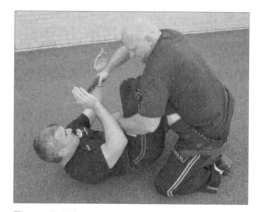

Figure 5.09b

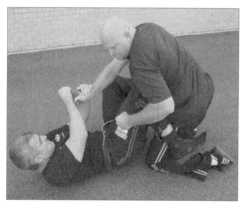

Figure 5.09c

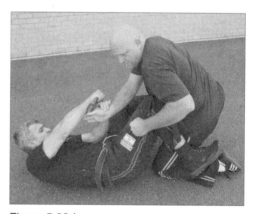

Figure 5.09d

Figures 5.09a–d. If the assailant successfully deploys the handgun from his waistband or elsewhere, the preferred defense is similar to the standing Gun Frontal Defense #2, using your farside arm to deflect-redirect while executing a body defense. Deflect-redirect the gun as soon as possible to clear your body from the line of fire. Using your opposite arm affords the best control of the handgun. To take away the handgun using Gun Frontal Defense #2, continue to "punch" through the handgun with your right arm and yank down on his gun-arm wrist with your left arm by cupping your hand.

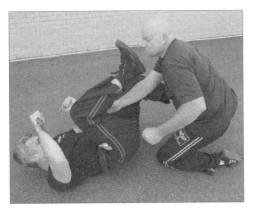

Figure 5.09e

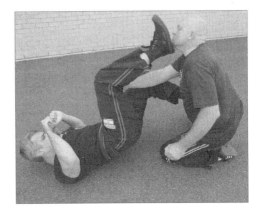

Figure 5.09f

Figures 5.09e–f. You can deliver strong heel kicks to his head. Another option is to establish firm and safe control over the barrel and use a scissors sweep, using your topside leg and bottom leg against base of his knee to turn the assailant onto his back where you can exert superior control over the weapon and remove the handgun from his grip. Be sure to control the barrel.

When You Are on Top

It is also possible that you will be fighting with an assailant with his back to the ground with you on top as he attempts to deploy a handgun.

This defense uses the same tactical principles and is more straightforward than the previous defenses covered when you are on your back. Again, the best defense is to prevent the assailant from successfully retrieving the weapon by disabling him with strikes or by using joint locks and pinning his gun-arm to his chest or to the ground while delivering withering combatives. If the assailant does successfully deploy the handgun, Frontal Defenses #1 or #2 may be used. Note: Frontal Defense #1 will require a slight modification in the handgun removal because you are on top of the assailant. As with the standing Frontal Defense #1, keep your weight on the handgun with simultaneous combatives to the head. Once you have debilitated the opponent, reach through to remove the handgun at the (internal) hammer; if necessary, use it in a cold weapon capacity, clear the weapon, put it back into battery, separate from the assailant, and create distance.

Handgun Defenses from the Side

Behind Your Arm

If an assailant threatens you with a handgun from your side and behind your arm, first turn your head around to recognize the threat. As with every other defense should you decide to react, calibrate the distance between you and the assailant. Again, be sure to turn your head to locate the handgun.

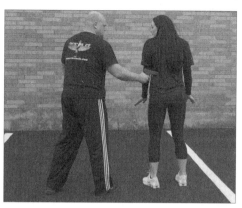

Figure 5.10a

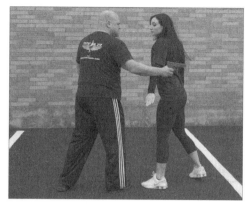

Figure 5.10b

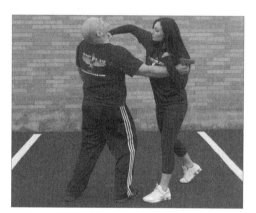

Figure 5.10c

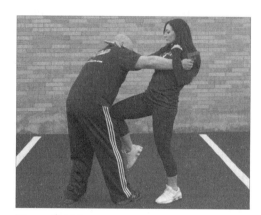

Figure 5.10d

Figures 5.10a–d. To defend, deflect and sweep aside the barrel using your left arm securing the handgun as previously covered in Figures 5.01u–zz. Use a sharp turn and pivot directly into the assailant with a punch to the face or throat strike. The arm leads the body. You could also strike the assailant in the groin with a punch, slap, or inverted palm-heel strike. Remember that a knee strike to the groin will lurch the assailant's body forward and you should use your free arm to brace his neck to prevent his inadvertently head-butting you. Never break contact with the assailant's gun-arm. Always and immediately secure the arm as close as possible to the gun holder's wrist to prevent the barrel being turning into you or being yanked back—which will be the attacker's instinctive response. Unlike the previous frontal defenses, you are not securing the gun by the barrel. Therefore, the handgun will remain functional until you remove it or it runs out of ammunition.

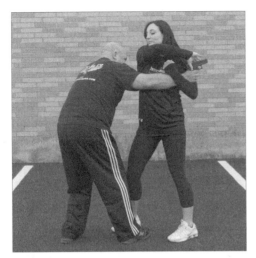

Figure 5.10e

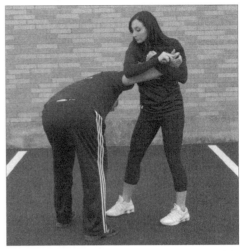

Figure 5.10f

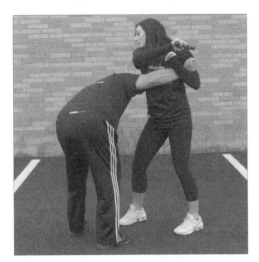

Figure 5.10g

Figures 5.10e–g. Once you have secured the gun-arm tightly with your arm wrapped as close to the assailant's wrist as possible, continue with your combatives until you neutralize the threat. After you have debilitated the opponent, maintain a strong vise on the assailant's gun-arm; take your free arm and cross it in front of your face reaching for the handgun's barrel. You should end up with your pinky toward the handgun's site. Grasp the gun strongly and turn it sharply about ninety degrees with the grip perpendicular to the ground to break the assailant's grip. The barrel should now be perpendicular to the gunman's hand. Once the grip is released, the trigger finger will still be in the handgun's trigger-well. Wrench the gun out likely breaking his trigger finger. You may then use the barrel of the gun to strike the opponent in the head. Again, note if you hit him in the temple, you risk killing him, so use only the force necessary to survive the situation.

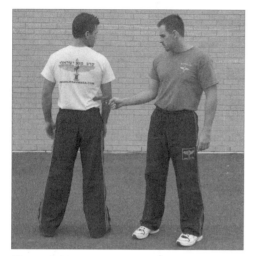

Figure 5.11a

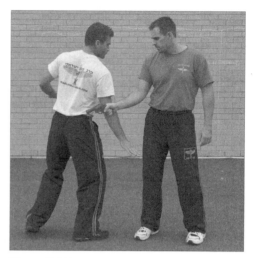

Figure 5.11b

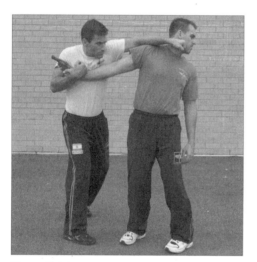

Figure 5.11c

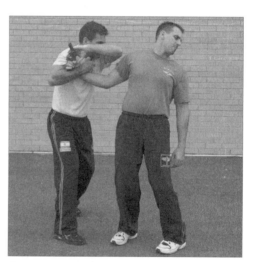

Figure 5.11d

Figures 5.11a–d. If the handgun is held close to your right arm or the right side of your back, a modification of this defense is to pivot in the opposite direction (the assailant's deadside) redirecting the gun while snaking your right arm around the assailant's gun-arm, and simultaneously delivering a punch to the chin, mandible, or temple, or fish-hook-eye gouge to the closest eye. In other words, this defense takes you to the outside of the assailant rather than to the inside as with the previous defense. You can continue with combatives with your free hand.

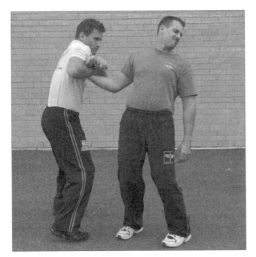 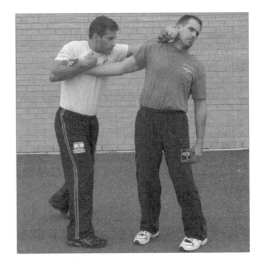

Figure 5.11e   Figure 5.11f

Figures 5.11e–f. To remove the weapon, use a modified grasp, ninety-degree wrist torque, proper takeaway angle to account for his trigger finger, and pry the handgun away.

In Front of Your Arm Variations

An assailant could hold the handgun to your side and in front of your arm making the disarm more challenging. This defense is used when your arms are down at your side and the assailant is facing in the same direction.

The Handgun is in Front of Your Arm and You Are Facing in the Same Direction as the Assailant

If the handgun is in front of your arm and you are facing in the same direction as the assailant, use a body defense and simultaneous deflection-redirection of the barrel to assert dominant weapon control and complete the disarm technique.

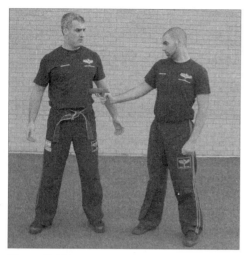

Figure 5.12a

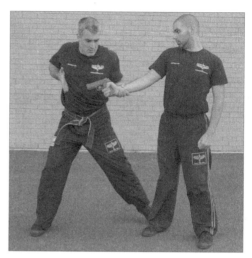

Figure 5.12b

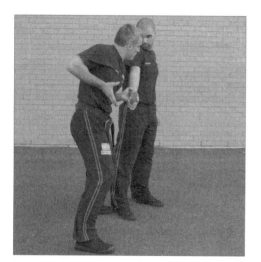

Figure 5.12c

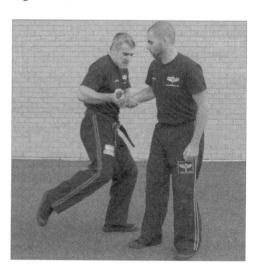

Figure 5.12d

Figures 5.12a–d. Take a small step backward and to the side at approximately a thirty-degree angle toward the assailant to clear the line of fire. As you step, simultaneously bring both arms up to your midsection with palms out and fingertips toward the ground. Your near arm will deflect the assailant's gun-arm away from you by deflecting-redirecting forward, and secure the wrist while your far arm is used to clasp the barrel and punch the gun away and out of his hands similar to Figures 5.07 h–l. Keeping both hands close to the midsection, pivot on the ball of your right foot toward the assailant to exert maximum disarming force.

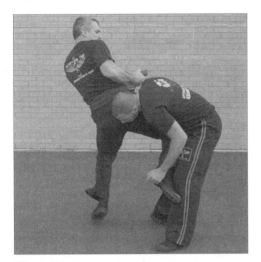

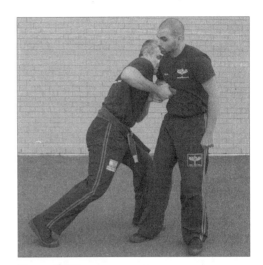

Figure 5.12e   Figure 5.12f

Figures 5.12e–f. To remove the weapon, a disarm option is to use a simultaneous knee strike to the groin or, alternatively, punch the barrel into his midsection targeting the liver as depicted in Figure 5.12f. Be sure to keep your torso and hand clear of the line of fire. You may also simply punch the barrel into the assailant's midsection including the liver. On hard contact with his torso, you can then elevate the barrel and use it for a modified uppercut strike to his jaw or throat followed by additional counterattacks.

The Handgun is in Front of Your Arm when Facing in the Opposite Direction as the Assailant

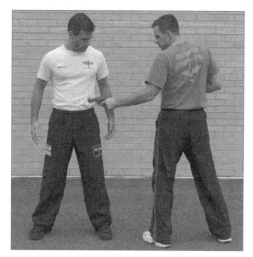

Figure 5.13a

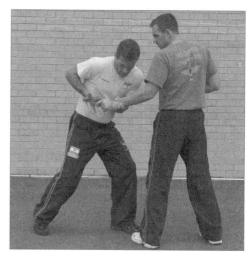

Figure 5.13b

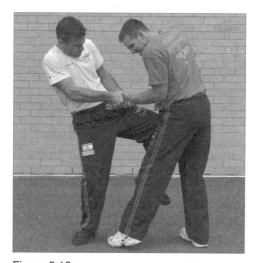

Figure 5.13c

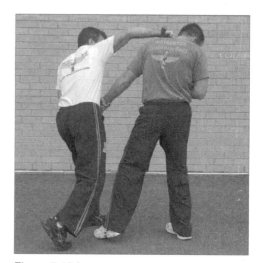

Figure 5.13d

Figures 5.13a–d. If the handgun is in front of your arm when facing in the opposite direction of the assailant, the defense remains the same with minor modification. Because the assailant has the handgun in his right hand with his left shoulder to the right of your torso, you will need to punch his wrist outward rather than inward. Perform the deflection-redirection with a simultaneous knee strike to the groin. Use the powerful momentum of the disarm and glicha (a sliding movement with your rear leg) to deliver a front knee into the assailant's groin. After the disarm, continue to use the handgun as a cold weapon followed by additional counterattacks.

The Handgun is in Front of Your Arm when Facing in the Opposite Direction when the Assailant is Farther Away.

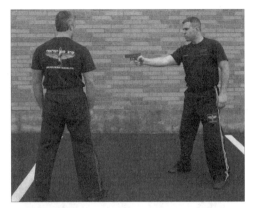

Figure 5.13e

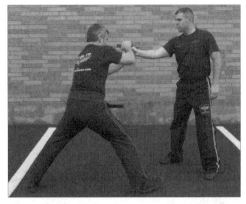

Figure 5.13f

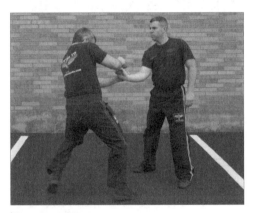

Figure 5.13g

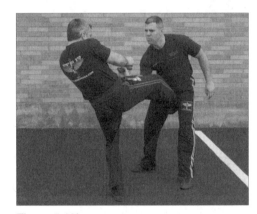

Figure 5.13h

Figures 5.13e–h. If the handgun is in front of your arm when facing in the opposite direction of the assailant, the defense is similar to Frontal Defense #2 with minor modification. If the assailant has the handgun in his right hand, using a subtle forward lean, punch out with your right hand to deflect and secure the handgun by the barrel simultaneously securing while blading your body and yanking down sharply on the assailant's gun-arm wrist with your left hand. Keep your left thumb attached to the hand in a "cupping motion." Forcibly punch the handgun through and away from the assailant's grip, jarring his gun-arm wrist down to remove the handgun. Be sure to use a simultaneous body defense to move to you off the line of fire. Deliver a straight kick to his groin with your right leg; then create distance to put the handgun back into battery. You also have the option of cold weapon combatives once you have deflected and punched the handgun out of the assailant's grip. Alternatively, close the distance and use the barrel to strike the assailant in the head or throat immediately after you confiscate it from his grip.

Handgun Defense Variations #1 and #2 Against / To the Side of the Head

Handgun in Front of the Ear

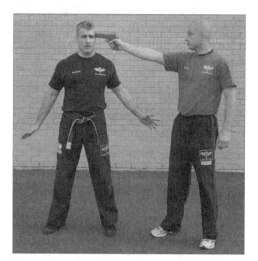

Figure 5.14a

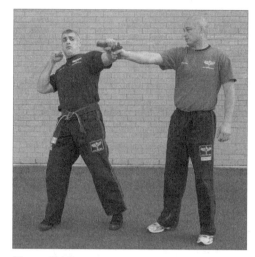

Figure 5.14b

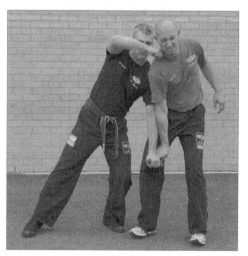

Figure 5.14c

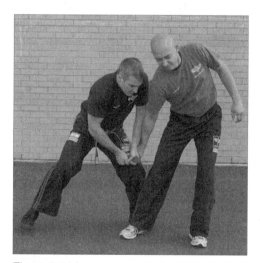

Figure 5.14d

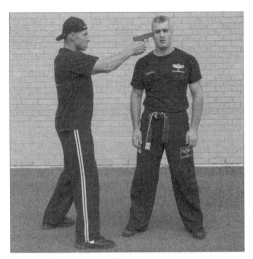

Figure 5.14e

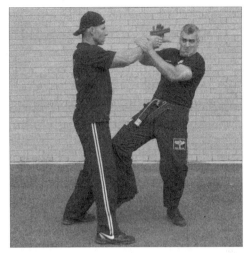

Figure 5.14f

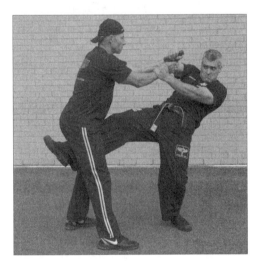

Figure 5.14g

Figures 5.14a–g. If an assailant holds a handgun to the side of your head in front of the ear, as with the other firearm defenses, deflect and control the barrel with a simultaneous body defense to clear the line of fire. The deflection-redirection, depending on which side the assailant is holding the gun, is a modification of Frontal Defense #1 or #2. For either modification, the head must move simultaneously in conjunction with the deflection-redirection away from the barrel. Do not swat the gun, but, rather, punch through it combined with lower body combatives. Remove the firearm using the same method as in Frontal Defense #1 and #2 respectively. Modified Frontal Defense #1 is best used against a right-handed assailant holding the handgun to the left side of your head with the barrel at or in front of your ear. Modified Frontal Defense #2 is optimally used against an assailant holding a handgun with his right hand to the right side of your head with the barrel at or in front of your ear.

Handgun Behind the Ear

If the handgun is held to the side of your head behind your ear, take your head off the line of fire by spinning into the attacker while simultaneously snaking your arm around the gun-arm for control. As you loop your arm around the gunman's arm, simultaneously punch him in the jaw, temple, or throat. You may also rake his eyes followed by additional retzev combatives and then remove the handgun as learned in Frontal Defense #1. A similar defense is represented in Figure series 5.20.

Hostage Defense Against a Handgun Held to the Side of Your Head

A gunman might hold you from behind with the handgun to the side of your temple and grip you with his other arm holding you hostage. The best solution, if feasible, is to comply and wait the situation out. If, however, you must react, krav maga provides a couple of solutions determined by the handgun barrel's placement in front or behind your ear. (Third-party hostage rescue techniques are in some ways similar, but a different subject matter.)

This seemingly grim situation may be defended in two ways. Realize that the assailant may have tight control over your movements with his arms wrapped around you and can sense your body shifts. If an assailant holds a gun to the side of your head and is behind you, as with the other gun defenses, deflect the barrel coupled with a simultaneous body defense to remove your head from the line of fire. There are two variations to this defense. Both involve a deflection-redirection and control technique using your farside arm. The specific defense is dictated by where the assailant places the barrel in relationship to your ear: (A) if the handgun is in back of your ear, deflect-redirect the barrel to the rear of your head; (B) if the handgun is front of your ear, deflect-redirect the barrel to the front of your head. Note: Variation B would be the same if a defender were placed on his knees with the handgun in front of his ear.

The first defense allows you to redirect the handgun with your farside arm while providing a subtle body defense to remove your head from the line of fire as you pin the handgun to the assailant's chest and secure his gun-arm.

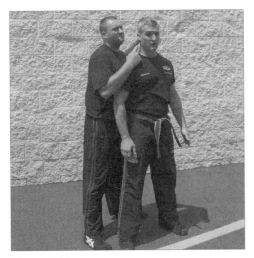

Figure 5.15a

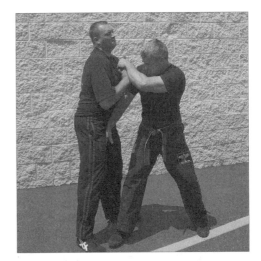

Figure 5.15b

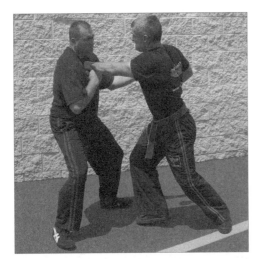

Figure 5.15c

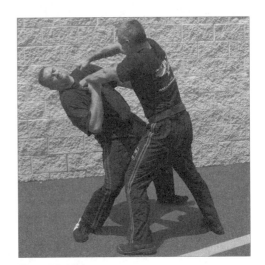

Figure 5.15d

Figures 5.15a–d. The deflection-redirection is similar to Handgun Frontal Defense #1. Your farside hand must lead the body as you spin into your assailant to control the handgun. Continue to turn deadside to properly control the handgun. You may also have the opportunity to strike him in the groin.

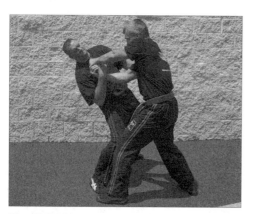

Figure 5.15e

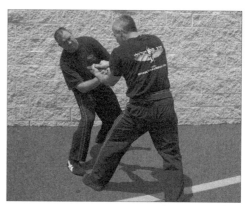

Figure 5.15f

Figures 5.15e–g. The follow-up disarm mirrors Frontal Defense #1.

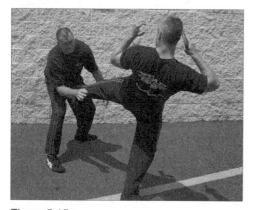

Figure 5.15g

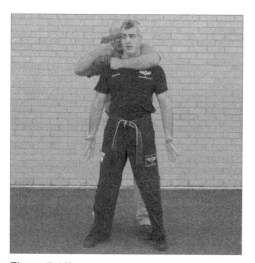

Figure 5.15h

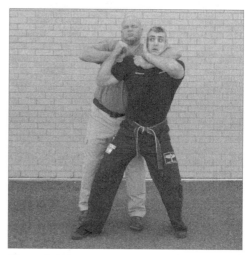

Figure 5.15i

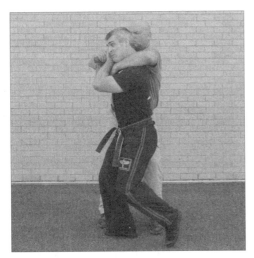

Figure 5.15j

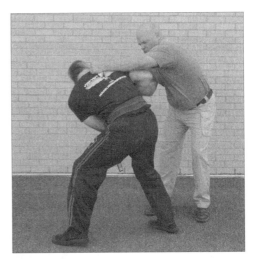

Figure 5.15k

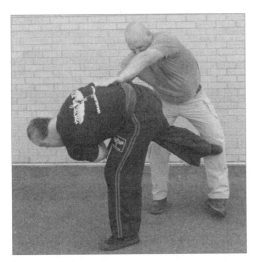

Figure 5.15l

Figures 5.15h–l. The second defensive option is available if the assailant has tight control over you with his free arm around your neck—hindering your ability to spin—and has the barrel placed in front of your ear or against your temple. Similar to the first option, use your far-side arm to deflect-redirect the barrel of the handgun. You must move your head backward to clear the line of fire while firmly snaking your hand up to clamp down on the barrel forcing it to turn away from you (optimally at ninety degrees). As you secure the barrel, immediately use your opposite hand to clamp down on the rear of the slide. Turn your body one-hundred-eighty degrees and pivot to remove the weapon debilitating him with a sidekick to his closest knee.

Hostage Defense Against a Handgun to the Side of Your Head When on Your Knees

A gunman might force you to kneel while positioning himself behind you with the handgun to the side of your temple in front of your ear, gripping you with his other arm holding you hostage. Again, the best solution, if feasible, is to comply and wait the situation out. If, however, you must react, krav maga provides the following solution.

This difficult position may be defended by deflecting-redirecting the handgun barrel to the outside while using your entire body to simultaneously turn against the wrist to wrest control, wrench away the handgun, and release his other hand as in Figures 5.15h–k. Realize again that the assailant may have tight control over your movements and can sense your body shifts. As always, deflect the barrel with a simultaneous body defense to remove your head from the line of fire. Secure the handgun immediately with your nearside arm while deflecting-redirecting the handgun sharply away from your head. Simultaneously slide your other arm across your body to secure the handgun at the rear. Rise up on your farside knee and, using a modified tsai-bake, turn sharply to your right at a ninety-degree angle to wrench the handgun away. You may also kick the assailant to disable him and then gain distance.

Defense While Lying in Bed Against an Assailant Holding a Handgun to Your Head

An intruder might hold a handgun to your head while awakening you in bed.

The same tactical principles apply; however, you might have covers or sheets on top of you, which obviously impede your movement. You must account for this in your movements. Handgun Defense #2 from the front is probably your best solution because it will divert the barrel toward the ceiling and afford you two-handed control of the weapon. Gravity, however, will be working against you, so maintain strong control of the barrel. Swing your legs around, if necessary, with the covers or sheets on top to deliver straight kicks to the assailant or to launch yourself from the bed to gain further control of the weapon and deliver combatives to subdue the assailant.

Handgun Defenses from the Rear

One of the most typical robbery scenarios is for an assailant to approach you from behind brandishing or indicating that he has a handgun.

If an assailant threatens you with a handgun from your rear, first turn your head around to recognize the threat. Try to recognize the position of both the assailant's hands.

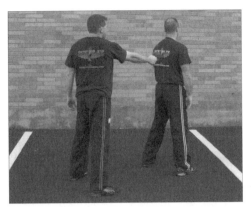

Figure 5.16a

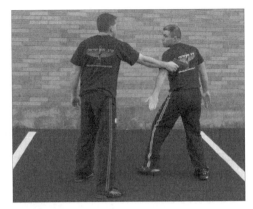

Figure 5.16b

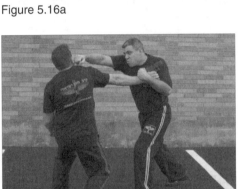

Figure 5.16c

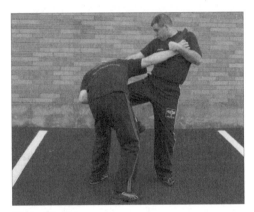

Figure 5.16d

Figures 5.16a–d. As with every other defense, should you decide to react, calibrate the distance between you and the assailant. Again, be sure to turn your head to locate the weapon. To defend, deflect and sweep aside the barrel snaking your left arm around the assailant's wrist, pulling it forcefully into the crook of your arm and shoulder. Take a sharp turn and pivot directly into the assailant with a punch to the face or throat strike. Note: You could also strike the assailant in the groin with a punch, slap, or inverted palm-heel strike, but a strong punch to the face is superior because your objective is to short-circuit his reaction process. If the assailant is using a two-handed grip, use an off-angle punch as your deflection-redirection. Knee combatives to the attacker's groin and thighs are strong follow-ups. Remember that a knee strike to the groin will lurch the assailant's body forward. Use your free arm to brace his neck to prevent his inadvertently head-butting you. Never break contact with the assailant's gun-arm.

Immediately and always secure the arm as close as possible to the gun holder's wrist to prevent the barrel being turned into you or being yanked back—which will be the attacker's instinctive response. Unlike the previous frontal defenses, you are not securing the gun by the barrel. Therefore, the handgun will remain functional until your remove it or it runs out of ammunition.

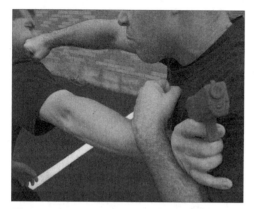

Figure 5.16e

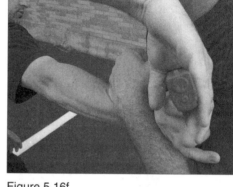

Figure 5.16f

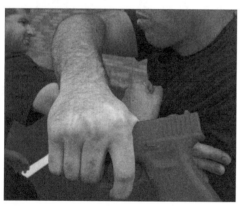

Figure 5.16g

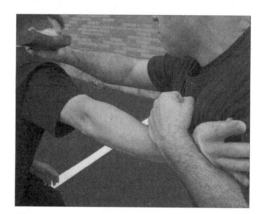

Figure 5.16h

Figures 5.16e–h. Once you have secured the gun-arm tightly with your arm wrapped as close to the assailant's wrist as possible, continue with your combatives until you neutralize the threat. After you have debilitated the opponent, maintain a strong vise on the assailant's gun-arm. Take your free arm and cross it in front of your face reaching for the handgun's barrel. You should end up with your pinky toward the handgun's site. Grasp the gun strongly and turn it sharply about ninety degrees with the grip perpendicular to the ground to break the assailant's grip. The barrel should now be perpendicular to the gunman's hand. Once the grip is released, the trigger finger will still be in the handgun's triggerwell. Wrench the gun out and away, which will likely break his trigger finger. You may then use the barrel of the gun to strike the opponent in the head. Again, note if you hit him in the temple, you risk killing him, so use only the force necessary to survive the situation.

If a gunman threatens you to the rear with a two-handed grip, the defense remains the same with the minor variation of ensnaring both of his arms. The disarm remains the same. If the handgun is held close to your right arm or the right side of your back, a modification of this defense is to pivot in the opposite direction (to the assailant's dead-side), redirecting the gun while snaking your right arm around the assailant's gun-arm, while simultaneously delivering a punch to the chin, mandible, or temple, or fishhook-eye gouge to the closest eye. In other words, this defense takes you to the outside of the assailant rather than to the inside as with the previous defense. You can continue with combatives with your free hand. To remove the weapon, use a modified grasp, ninety-degree wrist torque, and pry the handgun away.

Rear Handgun Defense with the Assailant Placing One Arm in Front to Push Forward or Keep His Distance

An assailant may threaten you from the rear with a handgun and try to push you forward with his free arm or simply use it as a buffer. His extended arm prevents you from using the previous defense from the rear. There are two defenses you can use.

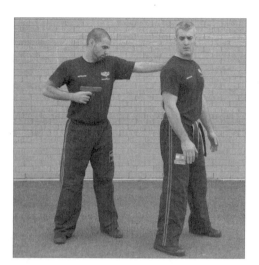

Figure 5.17a

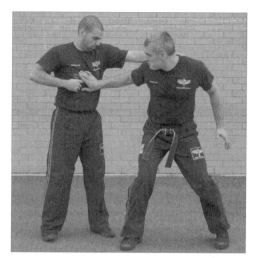

Figure 5.17b

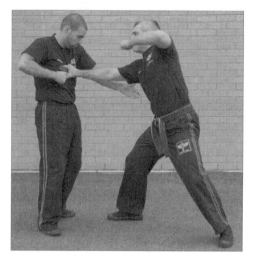

Figure 5.17c

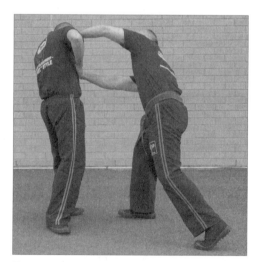

Figure 5.17d

Figures 5.17a–d. Again, for all threats to the rear, turn your head to see the threat. The first option is to swivel your head to the right to recognize the threat and discern if the distance is within your reach. Turn with your right shoulder into the assailant and use your left arm to deflect and pin the handgun to his chest while delivering simultaneous combatives. Be sure to make a deliberate sharp turn into the assailant with no wasted movement to redirect and control.

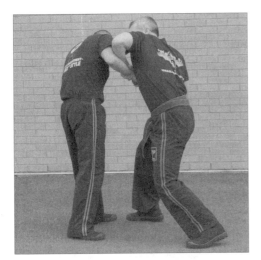

Figure 5.17e

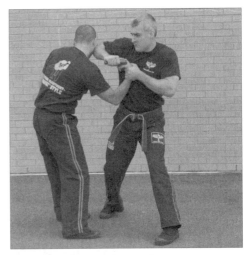

Figure 5.17f

Figures 5.17e–g. The handgun takeaway technique is a modification of the technique used when the handgun threat is to your side and in front of your elbow.

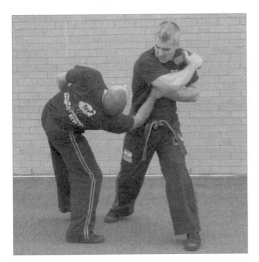

Figure 5.17g

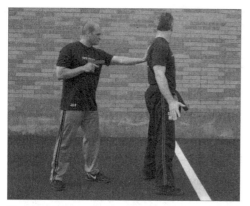

Figure 5.18a

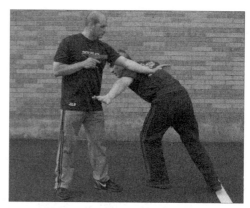

Figure 5.18b

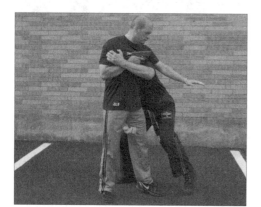

Figure 5.18c

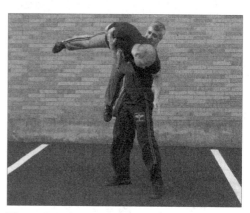

Figure 5.18d

Figures 5.18a–d. The second option involves a bucket-scoop takedown while simultaneously securing the handgun or gun-arm. The rear-gun-defense bucket scoop takes you to your opponent's deadside optimally pinning his firearm to his body with your left arm and shoulder while slamming your right forearm between his legs. As you strike and grab his testicles, position your hips slightly behind him to throw or dump him on his head. Pinning his arm will hinder his ability to break his fall. Sink your hips into your opponent and keep your back straight to load his weight properly. As with all throws, power emanates from your hips and core. Explode up through your legs keeping your back straight and head tucked, to avoid an elbow counterstrike from his free arm. The throwing motion loosely resembles pouring out a bucket, hence, the name.

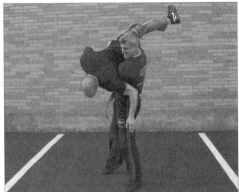

Figure 5.18e

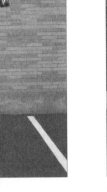

Figure 5.18f

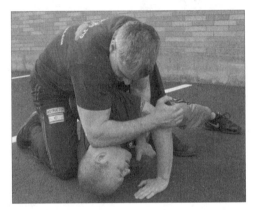

Figure 5.18g

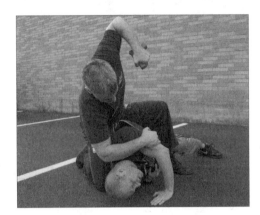

Figure 5.18h

Figures 5.18e–h. Continue to finish the defense by straddling him, delivering strikes to the back of his head or neck to prevent his turning on his back. When the threat is neutralized, carefully secure the weapon from underneath him. Pin the weapon to the ground and then forcefully rotate the barrel forty-five degrees to release his grip. Keep in mind the weapon is still in battery. When handling the handgun, be sure to apply firearm safety rules. Maintain strict control should he suddenly come to and try to use the firearm.

Rear Handgun Defense with Assailant's Free Arm on Your Shoulder for Control and Handgun Compressed against Your Torso

An assailant may threaten you from the rear with a handgun and place his free arm in on your shoulder to control you.

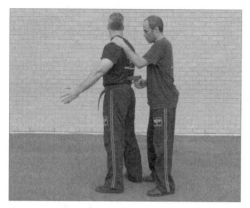

Figure 5.19a

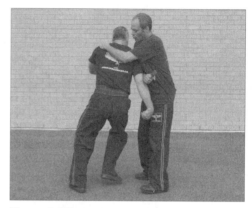

Figure 5.19b

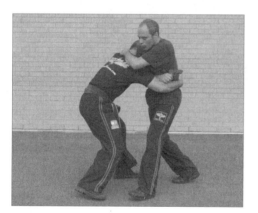

Figure 5.19c

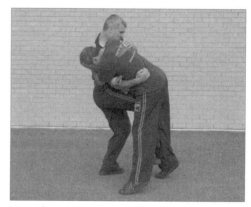

Figure 5.19d

Figures 5.19a–d. First, turn your head around to recognize the threat. To defend, deflect and sweep aside the barrel turning to your right redirecting-deflecting with your right arm, and using a sharp turn pivot directly into the assailant. As you turn, pin his gun-arm across his midsection forcing the barrel away from you. Simultaneously, deliver strong knees to his groin. Do not break contact with the assailant's gun-arm. To remove the handgun, remove your farside arm from his back and punch it away as depicted in Figures 5.07j–l.

Defense against a Handgun to the Back of the Head

The danger of being shot in the back of the head speaks for itself. An assailant holding a gun to the back of your head or pressed against it presents a challenging defense.

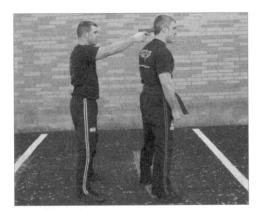

Figure 5.20a

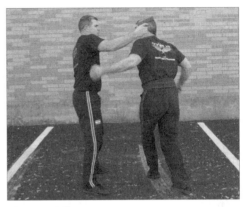

Figure 5.20b

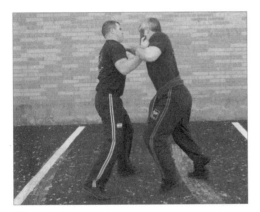

Figure 5.20c

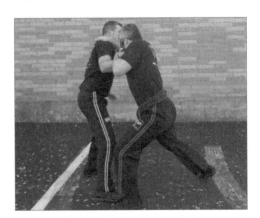

Figure 5.20d

Figures 5.20a–d. Use a body defense to remove your head from the line of fire while simultaneously spinning into the assailant to secure the weapon and close the distance. Always take the shortest path to clear the gun from your head (or any part of your body for that matter). In this defense, your head leads your body. The direction of your spin depends on which side of your head the barrel is held. Envision an imaginary line down the back of your skull. The handgun could be placed on this line, to the right or to the left of it. If the gun is held to right of your imaginary line, spin to your left following the same control method and a similar disarming tactic. Notably, a slight modification of this same defense would be used if a handgun were placed to the side of your head behind your ear (compare this variation to defending a handgun in front of your ear in Figures 5.14a–g.)

For example, regardless of which of the assailant's hands holds the handgun, if the handgun is held to left of your imaginary line, spin to your right to secure the gun with simultaneous combatives and complete the disarm.

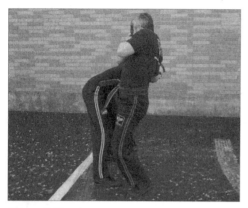

Figure 5.20e

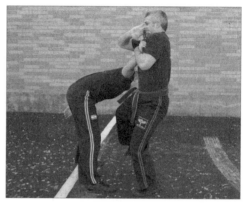

Figure 5.20f

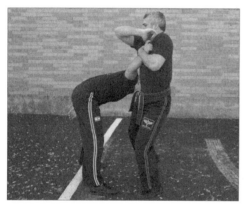

Figure 5.20g

Figures 5.20e–g. To secure the gun in either case, snake your nearside arm underneath the assailant's gun-arm and secure it firmly at the wrist to your upper pectoral muscle, while punching the assailant repeatedly in the neck or the head. You can also attack the eyes. Note: The handgun will likely fire and may continue to fire with deafening effect. You may also follow up with a shin kick to the groin or knee combative. Again, make sure the gun is securely pinned to your upper chest.

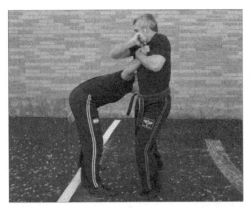

Figure 5.20h

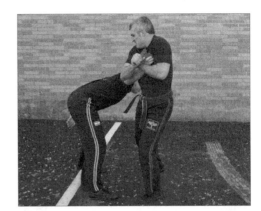

Figure 5.20i

Figures 5.20h–i. Once you have secured the gun-arm tightly with your arm wrapped as close to the assailant's wrist as possible (similar to the rear gun defense), proceed with the disarm as learned in Figures 5.16. You may wish to clasp the assailant's wrist with the cup of your hand and not a closed fist lock. Continue with your combatives until you neutralize the threat.

Handgun Defenses to the Back of the Head When Pressed Against a Wall

A gunman could force you to face a wall with a handgun pressed against or close to the back of your head with your hands placed against the wall. Obviously, the danger of being shot in the back of the head again speaks for itself.

Your Hands Are Pressed Against a Wall

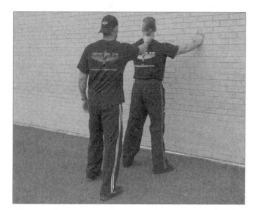

Figure 5.21a

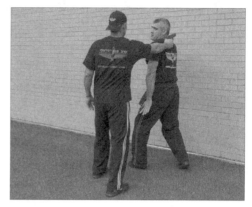

Figure 5.21b

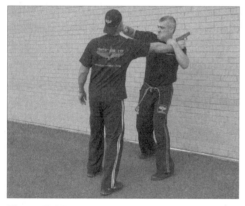

Figure 5.21c

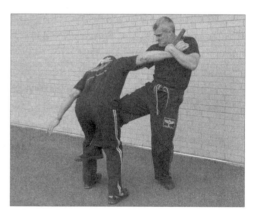

Figure 5.21d

Figures 5.21a–d. The defense against this threat differs slightly from the previous defenses in the specific tactics but not the overall strategy of deflecting-redirecting and counterattacking. As with all krav maga defenses, take the shortest route to clear the line of fire. Assess if the barrel is on the centerline of your skull or to the left or right of your centerline. Spin directly into the attacker's deadside (or liveside if necessary) while snaking your nearside arm to control the weapon and deliver combatives with your free arm and lower body. Remove the weapon as learned previously in Figures 5.07u–zz or 5.20d–j.

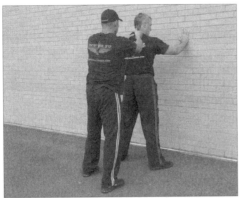

Figure 5.21e

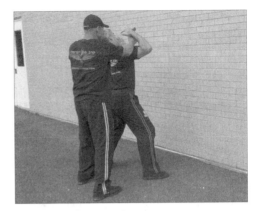

Figure 5.21f

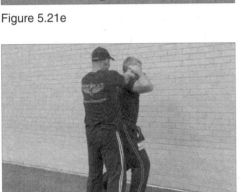

Figure 5.21g

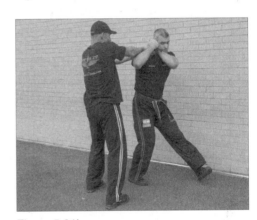

Figure 5.21h

Figures 5.21e–h. If your hands are against the wall with your arms extended out and the assailant has his free arm controlling you, spinning your head and moving into the assailant is *not* an option (as with the regular defense against a handgun threat to the back of the head). Your extended arms force you to spend more time in front of the barrel. Always keep in mind that the assailant will retract the weapon in an attempt to thwart a disarm attempt and maintain control. Therefore, rather than spin into the attacker for this defense, clear your head from the line of fire and redirect-control the weapon with your nearside hand. Most people are right-handed, so chances are you will move your head to your left while deflecting-redirecting with your right hand. Almost simultaneously with clearing your head from the line of fire and redirecting the barrel, bring your left hand across your face to cup the handgun at the hammer (internal or external). As soon as your other hand latches onto the handgun, continue to pivot and turn to your right to wrench the weapon away. As soon as opportune, use lower body combatives to neutralize the threat.

Handgun Defense from the Rear When the Assailant is Controlling/Choking You with His Free Arm

A gunman could hold you at gunpoint from the rear while to controlling-choking you with his free arm.

The defense against this threat is similar to the handgun defense from the rear (in Figures 5.20a–j) except that you must turn into the control/choke while snaking your nearside arm around the firearm.

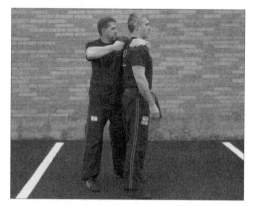

Figure 5.22a

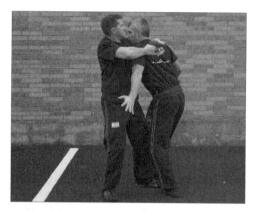

Figure 5.22b

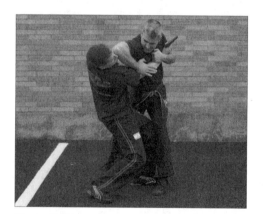

Figure 5.22c

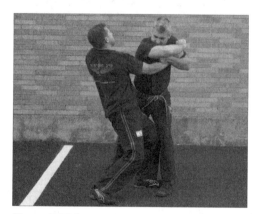

Figure 5.22d

Figures 5.22a–d. As you execute a simultaneous body defense and redirection, use your free arm to deliver an elbow strike or eye gouge. In this particular case, an over-the-top elbow strike can be highly effective. Note: A punch will also work as we emphasized in the rear defense when the gunman has his arm extended to your back. Be sure not take a wide arc. It is imperative that you burst deep into the assailant to take your head off the line of fire and close the distance. As you pivot, snake your left arm around the gunman's wrist and deliver strong combatives to his face.

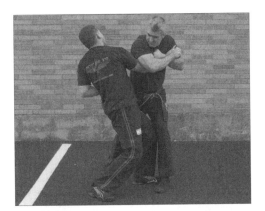

Figure 5.22e

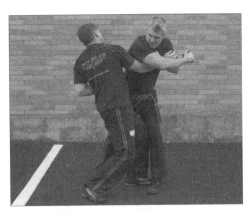

Figure 5.22f

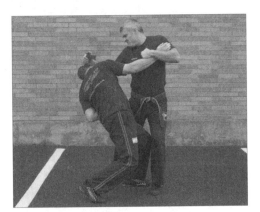

Figure 5.22g

Figures 5.22e–g. Remove the weapon using the handgun defense from the rear disarm technique similar to Figures 5.16.

Rear Handgun Defense to the Head When on Your Knees

A gunman could force you to your knees facing while away from him in what is commonly known as an execution position from the rear. Yet again, the danger of being shot in the back of the head speaks for itself and you must react immediately.

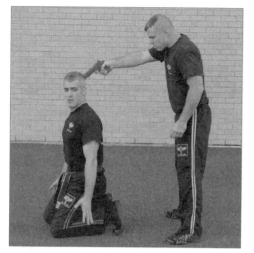

Figure 5.23a

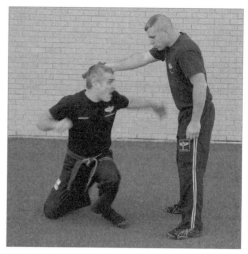

Figure 5.23b

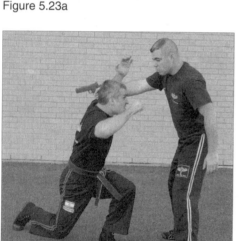

Figure 5.23c

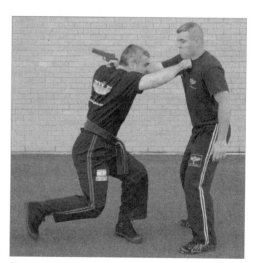

Figure 5.23d

Figures 5.23a–d. The defense against this threat is similar to the handgun defense from the rear except that you raise your left knee and sharply pivot on both balls of your feet to explode into the assailant. Do not take a wide arc. Pivoting on your knees must duplicate the "opening up" footwork used in the handgun defense from the rear (Figures 5.16). Similar to the handgun defense from the rear, if you decide to turn into the assailant to your left, turn one-hundred-eighty degrees by raising your left knee and spinning the ball of your right foot. It is imperative that you burst deep into the assailant to take your head off the line of fire and close the distance as he likely to retract the weapon.

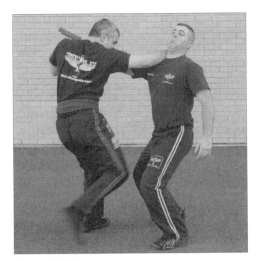

Figure 5.23e

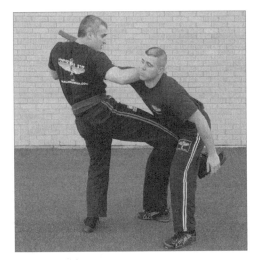

Figure 5.23f

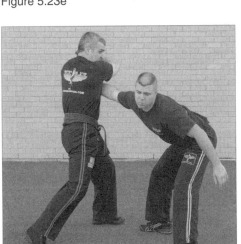

Figure 5.23g

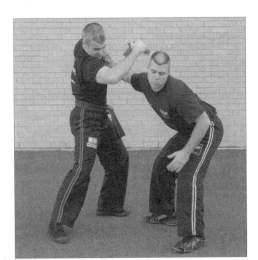

Figure 5.23h

Figures 5.23e–h. As you pivot, snake your left arm around the gunman's wrist and deliver strong combatives to his face; remove the weapon using the handgun defense from the rear disarm technique.

Sidearm Retention

Sidearm retention is a foremost concern for the law enforcement, military, and law-fully armed personnel. For sidearm retention, before the assailant can grab the defender's weapon, krav maga uses basic deflection-redirection defenses with a one-hundred-eighty-degree hip pivot to take the gun-side hip away while simultaneously striking or creating distance from the assailant. If the assailant successfully grabs the defender's holstered weapon, use the simultaneous defense and attack principle. With a typical Level 3- or 4-retention holster, the defender must secure the weapon with one of his forearms or his hands or by pressing against the top rear of the slide or grip. While securing the weapon, the defender must deliver combatives with his free arm, legs, and, possibly, head-butts. In the case of a tactical thigh rig, both hands may be needed to secure the weapon necessitating knee strikes or kicks while turning the gun leg away from the assailant while tucking the chin to protect the throat.

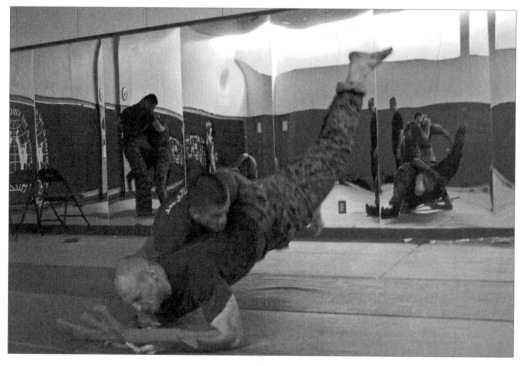

U.S. Marines training in Israeli krav maga. Photo courtesy of USMC Combat Camera.

CHAPTER 6

Rifle/Submachine Gun (SMG) Defenses

Frontal Rifle/SMG Defenses

Rifle/submachine gun (SMG) defenses from the front are similar in concept to handgun defenses but different in execution because of the firearm's length and operation.

Defending against a rifle/SMG threat utilizes the core krav maga principle of simultaneous weapon deflection-redirection and body defense movement combined with counterattacks. A distinct difference between a rifle/SMG design and a handgun is the firearm's length, especially if the rifle/SMG has an extended stock and an automatic fire capability. Certain SMGs such as the Uzi machine pistol might need to be defended against using the handgun defenses covered previously. Shotguns are also included in the rifle category for our discussion purposes. Keep in mind that a shotgun's discharge creates a wider berth of danger, as the shot scatters.

Krav maga's rifle/SMG defenses adapt to threats at different heights and angles. The following three frontal defense variations are also used to thwart a bayonet-type thrust attack. Practice each of these and decide which is most comfortable for you. Whichever defense you use, be sure to remain clear of the muzzle while controlling it. A semi-automatic or automatic rifle/SMG will continue firing as long as the gunman activates the trigger and the ammunition supply lasts. An automatic weapon can discharge thirty-plus rounds in just a few seconds. Keep in mind that these rounds also endanger third parties. Importantly, with rifle/SMG disarms, you are not interfering with the firing mechanism as some of krav maga's handgun defenses do.

Frontal Rifle/SMG Defense #1

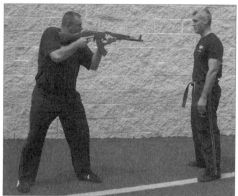

Figure 6.01a

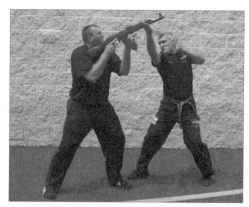

Figure 6.01b

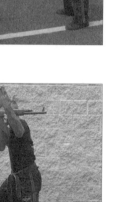

Figure 6.01c

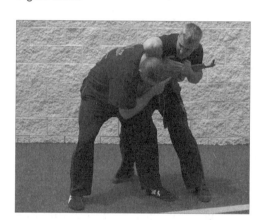

Figure 6.01d

Figures 6.01a–d. Frontal rifle/SMG Defense #1 uses a redirection of the rifle/SMG's barrel. As with all krav maga weapons defenses, the hand leads the body defense as you burst toward the weapon to close the distance. Extend your left arm out using the web of your hand to redirect the line of fire. Keep a slight bend in your elbow to prevent hyperextension of your elbow upon contact with the weapon. As soon as you deflect the barrel away, snake the opposite arm around the weapon's fore-grip to control it. As you move in, use opportune knee strikes to the assailant's lower body and/or elbows to the back of his head.

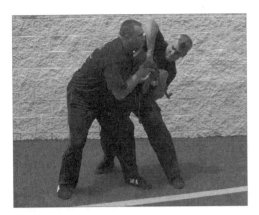

Figure 6.01e

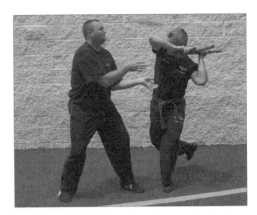

Figure 6.01f

Figures 6.01e–f. Reach over the assailant's shoulder and clench the rifle's butt stock (closest to the receiver). To remove the weapon, insert your right hand with the thumb pointed toward the ground to grasp the weapon's stock and yank the weapon toward you to weaken his leverage, and then yank sharply up. If the assailant has the stock tucked underneath his armpit, yank forward to dislodge it and then up. This removal technique may smash the assailant in the jaw as you remove the weapon. Note: If the stock is collapsed or retracted, cup your hand, and yank up at the rifle/SMG's pistol grip. If there is a two- or three-point sling attached, remove the sling by pulling it over the assailant's head in the direction of the under-slung arm. In other words, take the sling over his shoulder toward the sling's loop under his armpit. Wrench the weapon away and use it for further combatives, or turn it on the assailant if it is still in battery.

Another control option is to exert dominant control over the assailant's head to wrench his neck back while maintaining strict control of the muzzle to take him down to the ground for weapon removal. If the assailant uses a right-handed grip on the weapon, move to his left side to peel the weapon out from underneath him. (If he is holding the weapon in his left hand, go to the right side.)

Frontal Defense #1 from an Execution Position

As discussed with the previous handgun defense from your knees depicted in Figures 5.06, try not to go to your knees. If you must comply and then react, here is the preferred technique.

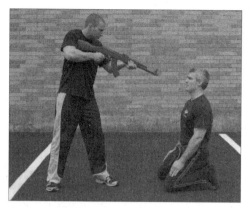

Figure 6.01g

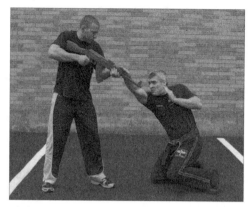

Figure 6.01h

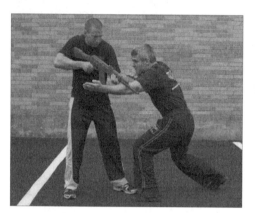

Figure 6.01i

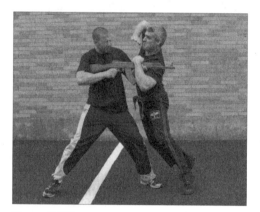

Figure 6.01j

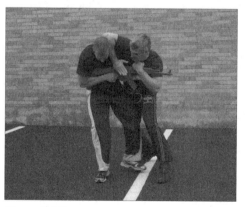

Figure 6.01k

Figures 6.01g–k. This series is a modification of the defense if you found yourself on your knees with a rifle/SMG pointed at your midsection as demonstrated in the following Figures 6.02g–l.

Frontal Rifle/SMG Defense #2 to the Deadside

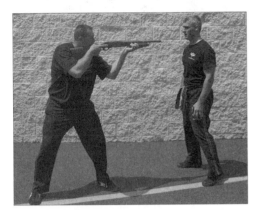

Figure 6.02a

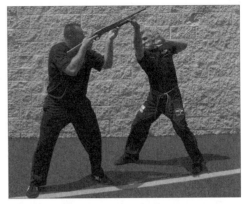

Figure 6.02b

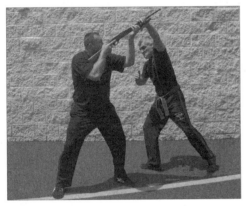

Figure 6.02c

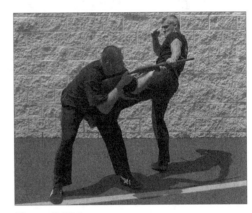

Figure 6.02d

Figures 6.02a–d. Rifle/SMG frontal Defense #2 is similar to rifle/SMG frontal Defense #1 except the weapon is seized and controlled differently. This particular defense has merit if the rifle/SMG is pointed to your midsection as demonstrated in Figures 6.02h–j. To clear the line of fire, the hand leads the body using a slight body defense and then sidestep to your right. By extending your right arm, use the web of your hand to redirect the line of fire. Again, keep a slight bend in your elbow to prevent hyperextension upon contact with the weapon. As soon as the initial deflection-redirection is made, switch control of the weapon to your left hand while simultaneously delivering a straight or roundhouse kick (depending on your position) to the assailant's groin with the ball of your foot. If for some reason you missed the switch of your right hand to your left hand to control the muzzle, close the distance snaking your left arm around the barrel and delivering combatives with the right arm similar to rifle/SMG frontal Defense #1.

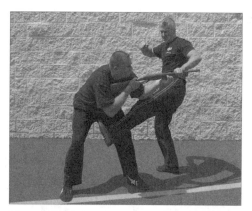

Figure 6.02e

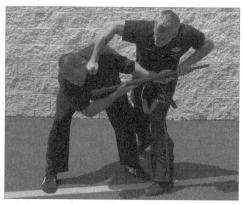

Figure 6.02f

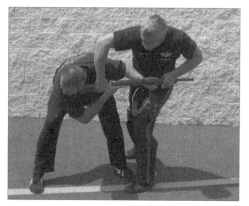

Figure 6.02g

Figures 6.02e–g. Proceed with straight punches using your right arm, optimally landing the punch as your left foot touches the ground for maximum momentum and efficacy of movement. The same defense may be used if a rifle/SMG is pointed at your midsection. Remove the long gun as depicted in Figures 6.01.

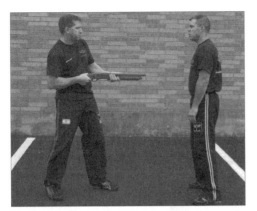

Figure 6.02h

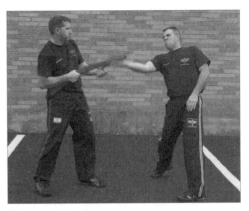

Figure 6.02i

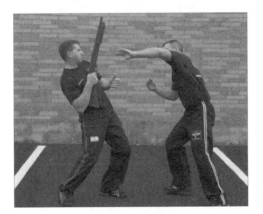

Figure 6.02j

Figures 6.02h–j. A mid-level defense is performed in the same manner as depicted in Figures 6.02.

Lastly, in rifle/SMG defenses to the front, you may use a variation of Frontal Handgun Defense #1 deflecting-redirecting the barrel to pin it to the gunman's chest while delivering simultaneous counterattacks. However, this defense is less preferred. The danger is that the assailant has superior leverage because of the rifle/SMG's length and his two-handed grip to either wrench it away from you even while you counterattack or he can use the rifle/SMG butt to counterattack you. The muzzle may also be hot from previous firing or can quickly become hot as the weapon discharges. Nevertheless, a modified Frontal Handgun Defense will work, but the rifle/SMG's removal will differ. Exert strong control over the barrel because the gunman has the advantage of two hands and leverage to wrest it from your grip. Your combatives must very strong to debilitate him and move with him as you pummel him backward.

Frontal Rifle/SMG Defense #3 to the Liveside

This defense may be necessary when you are positioned closer to the assailant's liveside and must proceed accordingly.

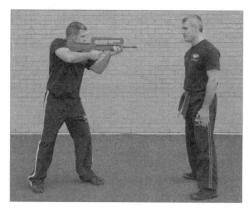

Figure 6.03a

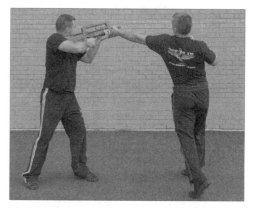

Figure 6.03b

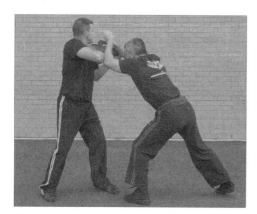

Figure 6.03c

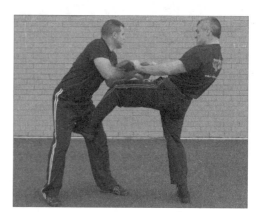

Figure 6.03d

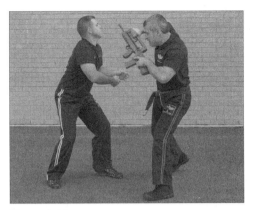

Figure 6.03e

Figures 6.03a–e. Frontal rifle/SMG Defense #3 also involves a redirection of the rifle/SMG's barrel. The hand again leads the body defense as you deflect-redirect the muzzle and burst toward the weapon closing the distance to the assailant's liveside. Again, keep in mind the weapon will keep discharging if the assailant has the trigger depressed as long as ammunition supplies last. As soon as the initial deflection-redirection is made, close the distance to the assailant by thrusting both of your forearms with the fleshy side toward the weapon. Continue to close the distance and forcefully drive the undersides of your forearms into the weapon to prevent a follow-up horizontal attack or "butt swing." After making contact with your forearms, use your hands in a claw-like cup to rake down on the weapon and turn the top of the weapon ninety degrees toward you while wrenching it from the assailant's grip. Deliver a simultaneous straight knee or kick to the assailant's groin. In other words, when removing the automatic weapon, be sure to turn the magazine into the gunman. This move serves the dual purpose of disengaging his grip from the weapon and allowing an unimpeded straight knee or kick counterattack with no potential injury from the magazine. If the rifle/SMG has a two- or three-point sling attached, remove the sling as depicted in Figures 6.04. You may also use the weapon, especially the magazine, for combatives against the assailant's face prior to fully removing the weapon. Wrest the weapon away by yanking back sharply.

Bayonet/Sharp-Elongated Weapon Defenses

Bayonet/sharp-elongated weapon defenses are similar to long-gun defenses by design—reinforcing krav maga's fundamental principle of learning a few core defenses to apply against a variety of attacks.

Krav maga's bayonet defenses derive from its rifle/SMG frontal defenses. The two primary bayonet defense variations parallel frontal rifle/SMG Defenses #2 and #3 respectively.

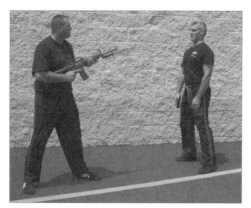

Figure 6.04a

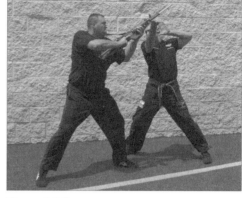

Figure 6.04b

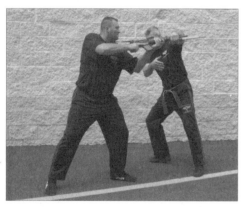

Figure 6.04c

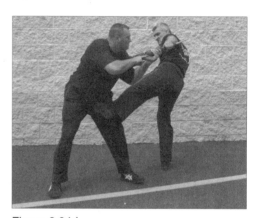

Figure 6.04d

Figures 6.04a–d (Liveside). The hand leads the body using a slight body defense The hand leads the body using a slight body defense and taking a deep forty-five degree step to your right placing you to the assailant's liveside. This is important because he will likely retract the weapon upon your deflection; you must close the distance to secure it. As soon as the initial deflection-redirection is made, switch control of the weapon to your left hand while simultaneously delivering a straight or roundhouse kick (depending on your position) to the assailant's groin with the ball of your foot. If for some reason you missed the switch of your right hand to your left hand to control the muzzle, close the distance snaking your left arm around the barrel and delivering combatives with the right arm similar to rifle/SMG front Defense #1.

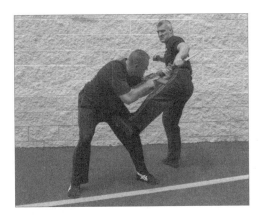

Figure 6.04e

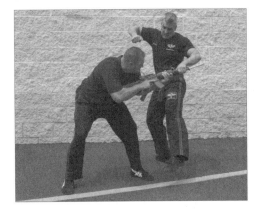

Figure 6.04f

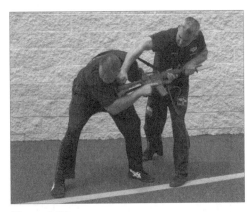

Figure 6.04g

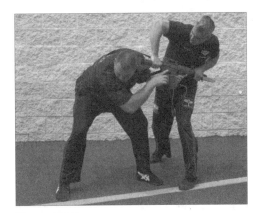

Figure 6.04h

Figures 6.04e–h. Follow up with straight punches using your right arm, optimally landing the punch as your left foot touches the ground for maximum momentum and efficacy of movement. Do not let go of the weapon under any circumstances.

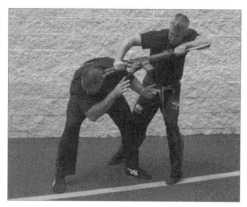

Figure 6.04i

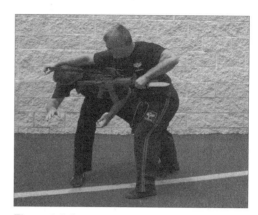

Figure 6.04j

Figures 6.04i–j. Use the weapon as a cold combative. To remove the weapon, proceed with weapon removal as learned in rifle/SMG Defense #1 removing the sling from over the top of his head.

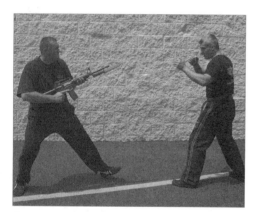

Figure 6.04k

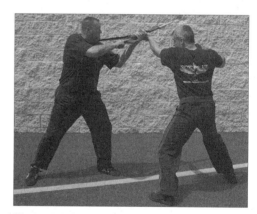

Figure 6.04l

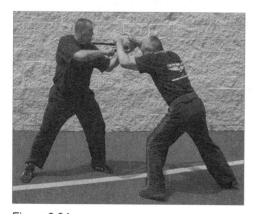

Figure 6.04m

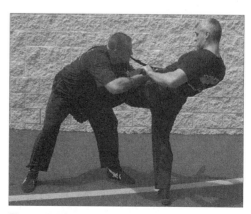

Figure 6.04n

Figures 6.04k–n. This bayonet defense option also involves a redirection of the rifle/SMG's barrel. The hand again leads the body as you deflect-redirect the muzzle and burst toward the weapon closing the distance to the assailant's liveside. As soon as the initial deflection-redirection of the bayonet is made, close the distance to the assailant by thrusting both of your forearms with the fleshy side toward the weapon. Continue to close the distance and forcefully drive the undersides of your forearms into the weapon to prevent a follow-up horizontal attack or butt swing. After making contact with your forearms, use your hands in a claw-like cup to rake down on the weapon and turn the top of the weapon ninety degrees toward you wrenching it from the assailant's grip. Deliver a simultaneous straight knee or kick to the assailant's groin. In other words, when removing the automatic weapon, be sure to turn the magazine into the gunman. This move serves the dual purpose of disengaging his grip from the weapon and allowing an unimpeded straight knee or kick counterattack with no potential injury from the magazine. You may also use the weapon, especially the magazine, for combatives against the assailant's face prior to fully removing the weapon, especially if a sling is attached. After disabling the assailant, you can remove the sling by slipping it over the top of the assailant's head. If he falls backward with the weapon while it is still slung, hold onto the weapon and step to his side to avoid being pulled on top of him.

Building on the two previous options, two additional variations enable you to choke the attacker.

As with frontal rifle/SMG defenses #2 and #3, these two variations redirect the weapon combined with a clothesline combative (arimi) into a choke. The difference is which arm you use to deflect the weapon, which, in turn, determines if you will step to the attacker's liveside or deadside. In either variation, as soon as the initial deflection-redirection is made, your other arm delivers a strike to the opponent's throat and then you step through for a choke.

Keep your striking arm slightly bent to prevent your elbow from hyper-extending your elbow. Maintaining contact, step around the opponent securing his neck in the crook of your arm. Cinch the choke with your hand and thrust your hips into the attacker lifting him from the ground positioning and loading your hips properly. These technique variations are only to be used in a life and death situation.

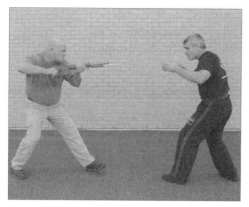

Figure 6.05a

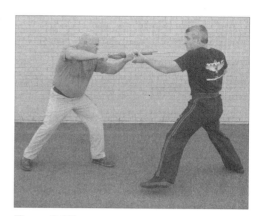

Figure 6.05b

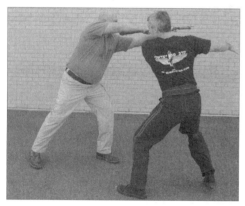

Figure 6.05c

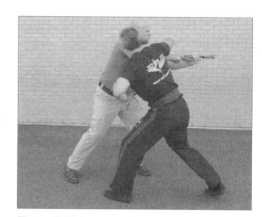

Figure 6.05d

Figures 6.05a–d. Bayonet defense to the liveside using arimi, a clothes-line strike.

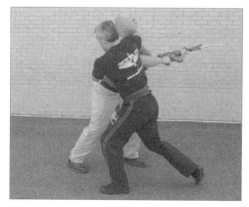

Figure 6.05e

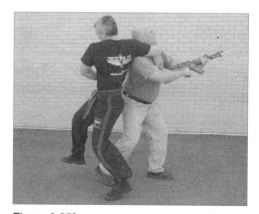

Figure 6.05f

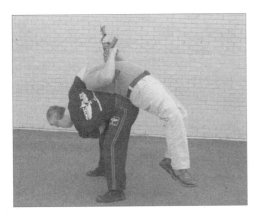

Figures 6.05e–g. Complete the liveside defense with a choke.

Figure 6.05g

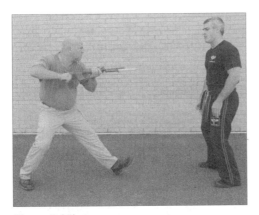

Figure 6.05h

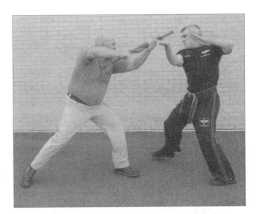

Figure 6.05i

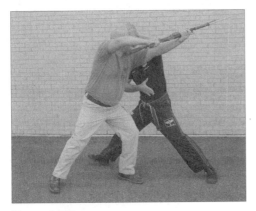

Figure 6.05j

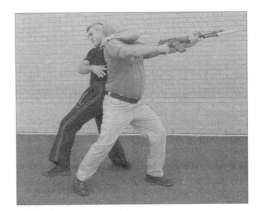

Figure 6.05k

Figures 6.05h–k. Bayonet defense to the deadside using arimi.

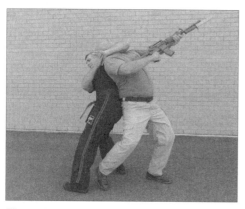

Figure 6.05l

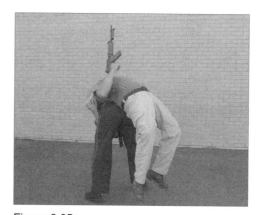

Figure 6.05m

Figures 6.05l–m. Complete the deadside defense with a choke.

Bayonet-Type Stab with the Defender on His Back

A standing attacker could try to stab a defender with an elongated weapon such as a bayonet or spear. You must redirect the weapon with your nearside hand while turning onto your hip to use a slight body defense.

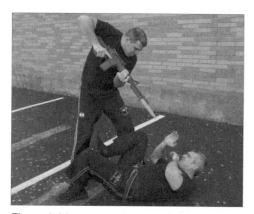

Figure 6.06a

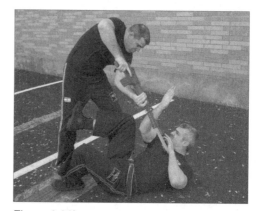

Figure 6.06b

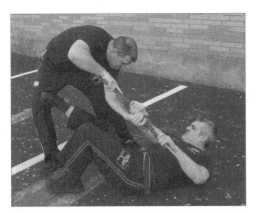

Figure 6.06c

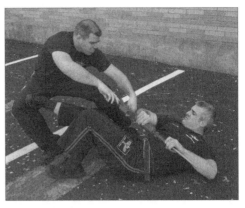

Figure 6.06d

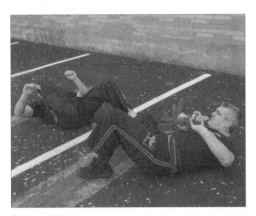

Figure 6.06e

Figures 6.06a–e. If you were on your back defending against an elongated weapon thrust, you may use a modified L block (similar to the straight stab defense in Figures 4.04) to deflect the weapon while transitioning to control the weapon similar to the previous rifle/SMG defenses. To counterattack, use your nearside leg to kick and buckle the attacker's knee while maintaining strict control of the weapon. Do your best to secure it with both hands, as the attacker will likely yank the weapon back in an attempt to stab you again. Lastly, if your timing is correct and your leg is in position, you might deflect the firearm away with your leg to then kick the attacker in his knees and transition to your feet immediately to finish the defense.

Rifle/SMG Defenses from the Rear

To defend against a rifle/SMG threat to your rear, you may use a defense similar to a handgun threat from the rear to deflect-redirect and secure the barrel while spinning deep into the gunman's deadside using strikes to disable and crumple him to the ground. You may also use a "bucket scoop" takedown pinning him to the ground on top of his rifle/SMG.

If an assailant threatens you with a rifle/SMG from your rear, turn your head around to recognize the threat. As with every defense, should you decide to react, calibrate the distance for the disarm. The preference is to move to the assailant's deadside. Note: If the gunman points the barrel at the left or right side of your back, the defense can also be performed to the assailant's liveside.

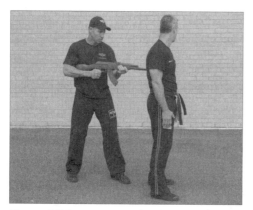

Figure 6.07a

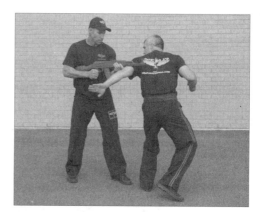

Figure 6.07b

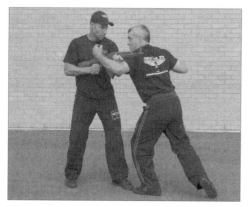

Figure 6.07c

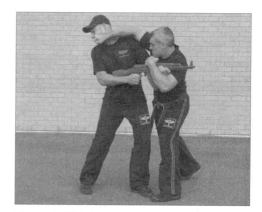

Figure 6.07d

Figures 6.07a–d. For Rifle/SMG Rear Defense #1 to the deadside, the head leads the body to recognize the threat, deflect-sweep aside the barrel using your left arm while firmly to snaking it around the barrel to secure it. Pivot sharply and directly into the assailant to place you on his deadside. Simultaneously secure the barrel in the crook of your elbow to prevent the muzzle from being turned back into you. Pinning the rifle/SMG to your torso, immediately punch him in the head. Continue your combatives until the gunman is no longer a threat and you have control of the weapon similar to Figures 6.01a–f.

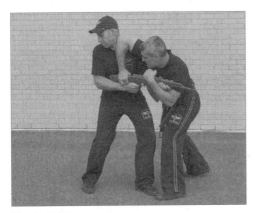

Figure 6.07e

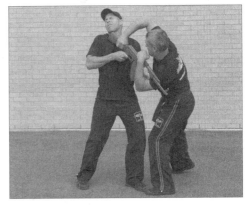

Figure 6.07f

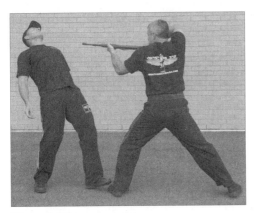

Figure 6.07g

Figures 6.07e–g. After you have debilitated the gunman, maintain a strong vise grip on the fore-grip with the crook of your elbow, and take your free arm to grip the smallest part of the stock closest to the gunman's trigger hand. Yank the stock toward you and sharply up, redirecting the barrel into the gunman.

A three-point sling will force you to remove the rifle/SMG by keeping the barrel firmly entrenched in the crook of your elbow and using your free hand to slip the sling over his head. Recognize which arm is under-slung for proper removal. A third option is to use the sling to choke the gunman.

Bucket Scoop Takedown Rifle/SMG Defense from the Rear

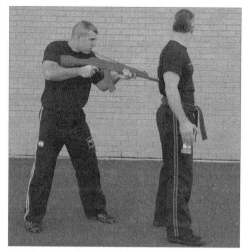

Figure 6.08a

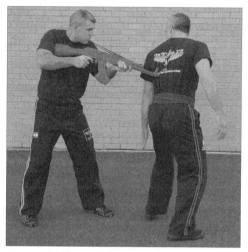

Figure 6.08b

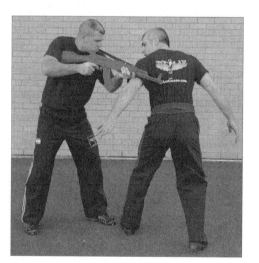

Figure 6.08c

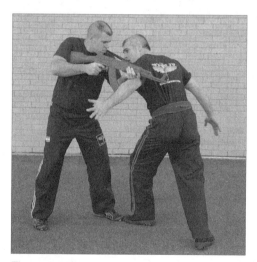

Figure 6.08d

Figures 6.08a–d. Another option using the same directional turn (pivoting to your left as in the previous Figures 6.07a–g) is to use the bucket scoop forgoing other combatives to drop the gunman on his head as previously covered in the rear handgun defense (Figures 5.18).

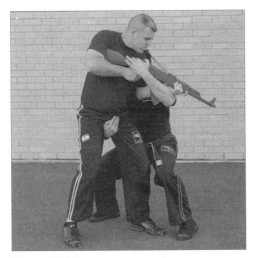

Figure 6.08e

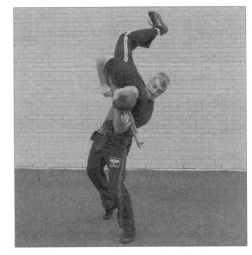

Figure 6.08f

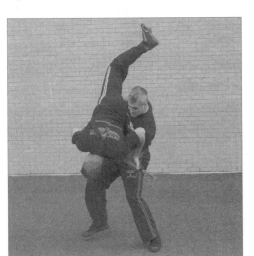

Figure 6.08g

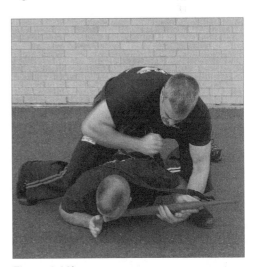

Figure 6.08h

Figures 6.08e–h. Firmly pin the rifle/SMG to the gunman's chest just forward of the magazine-well. Remember, the rifle/SMG will remain functional until you remove it. The rear-gun-defense bucket scoop takes you to your opponent's deadside securing him around his torso or optimally pinning his gun-arm to his body forcing the muzzle outward with your left arm and shoulder while slamming your right forearm between his legs. As you strike or grab his testicles, position your hips slightly behind him to throw or dump him on his head. Pinning his arm will hinder his ability to cushion his fall. Sink your hips into your opponent and keep your back straight to load your hips properly. As with all krav maga throws, power emanates from your hips and core. Explode up, keeping your back straight and head tucked, to avoid an elbow counterstrike from his free arm. The throwing motion loosely resembles pouring out a bucket, hence, the name. Finish the defense by delivering strikes to the back of his neck.

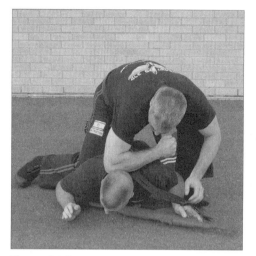

Figure 6.08i

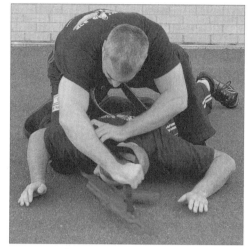

Figure 6.08j

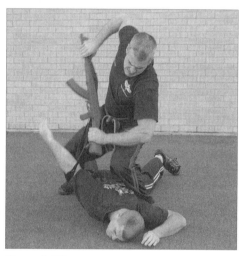

Figure 6.08k

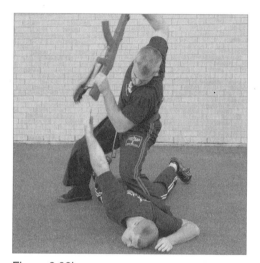

Figure 6.08l

Figures 6.08i–l. Only when the threat is neutralized should you secure the weapon from underneath him. Of course, when handling the firearm be sure to apply all rifle/SMG safety rules when removing the weapon.

Rifle/SMG Defenses from the Rear with One Hand on the Weapon and the Other Hand Extended in Front

This defense mirrors the rear handgun and rifle/SMG defenses you have already learned. An assailant may threaten you from the rear with a rifle/SMG and place his free arm in front of him and to your back as a buffer to keep his distance. He may try push you forward with his free arm. His extended arm prevents you from using the previous defense from the rear. There are two defenses you can use.

Turn your head to see the threat. The first option involves the sharp body defense turn to the deadside and bucket scoop takedown simultaneously securing the rife/SMG usually at the magazine insertion point demonstrated in Figures 6.08. After your takedown, continue to finish the defense by delivering strikes to the back of his neck. Only when the threat is neutralized should you roll the assailant over making sure to roll his back away on the side of the stock (not the muzzle side) so that you can maintain control should he suddenly come to and try to use the firearm. Of course, when handling the rifle/SMG, all firearm safety rules apply.

The second less preferred option is to swivel your head to the right, then turn with your right shoulder into the assailant, and use your right arm to deflect and pin the rifle/SMG to his chest with one or both of your arms while delivering simultaneous combatives as shown in Figures 5.17 with a handgun. Be sure to make a deliberate sharp turn into the assailant with no wasted movement to redirect and control. The rifle/SMG takeaway technique is the same as the Frontal Defense #1 from the front.

Defense Against a Rifle/SMG from the Rear While Being Pushed with the Free Arm

An assailant may threaten you from the rear with a rifle/submachine gun (SMG) and try to push you forward with his free arm. This defense is similar to defending against a handgun when an assailant has his free arm extended to your rear to create distance demonstrated in Figures 5.18 against a handgun threat. This extremely potent takedown defense allows you to strike the opponent's groin from the rear while dropping him face down onto the ground pinning him with the rifle/SMG.

If timed properly, you can use the assailant's push to your advantage. This bucket-scoop defense simultaneously secures the rifle/SMG and requires excellent timing. Turn your head to see the threat. The rear-gun-defense bucket scoop takes you to your opponent's deadside as learned in Figures 5.18.

Rifle/SMG Defenses from the Side

Rifle/SMG defenses from the side follow the same principles as handgun defenses found in Figures 5.11, 5.12, 5.13, and 5.14; however, the long gun's control and removal is different. Use the same removal as covered in the rifle/submachine gun (SMG) rear defense (Figures 6.07).

Rifle/SMG Weapon Retention

Rifle/SMG retention, with or without a sling, uses the simple concept of turning the assailant's force against him as he attempts to wrest the weapon away. By moving in the direction of the weapon pull, the defender's momentum increases the power and effectiveness of the strikes. Importantly, the rifle/SMG underside is turned toward the assailant to break his grip while turning the magazine outward clears the way for kicks and knee counterstrikes along with a possible strike with the weapon.

Note: If someone has a hot weapon, use weapon retention/cold combatives and then go hot.

CHAPTER 7

Kravist Weapon Defense Drills

Working with a good partner to practice and perfect weapon defense techniques is instrumental to your development as a kravist. The force and speed of the mock attacks should be gradually built up over time as your defensive skill sets improve. We do not advocate training with real weapons. Facsimile training weapons are readily available. We highly recommend BLUEGUNS® (www.blueguns.com) facsimile weapons for your training needs. Rubber or plastic knives and padded batons can also be acquired through Asian World of Martial Arts (www.awma.com). Eye protection, especially when training against edged-weapons attacks is prudent and always a must when practicing disarms with projectile-firing facsimile firearms.

Training Drills with a Partner

As you work with a partner, you will develop trust enhancing your ability to work with one another and enabling you to "go harder" as you progress within your respective skill sets. Training with multiple partners is also beneficial for the obvious reason that no two people move exactly alike. Someone with longer limbs will execute attacks and defenses differently than someone with shorter limbs. Bodyweight and strength are also highly influential training factors. Men and women should train with one another interchangeably. Coordinate your training with your partner or group of partners to ensure maximum training benefit. Designate who will perform the specific technique against the corresponding mock attack. After sufficient practice and familiarity with a given technique, series of techniques, and the overall training concept, introduce variations.

Training scenarios and variations with a partner should be worked in two practice phases: (1) *limited*—where you predetermine how your partner will attack and vary the designated attacks; (2) *unlimited*—you know an attack will come, but not what type or when. Limited training technique, for example, might include practicing defenses against pre-set overhead stab attacks. You know your partner is going to attack with an edged weapon slamming it overhead and down into your neck area. Following this limited training method, your partner at the direction of an instructor or his own initiative, will inform you that he will throw a right hook stab to your head. The point is that you know what is coming.

Unlimited open training allows your training to encompass the entire scope of weapon attack variations. Unlimited open training is used at the most advanced levels to resemble the street's unexpected dangers. Therefore, your partner could have any weapon in his hand or no weapon at all. Using the above example of an overhead-stab limited training exercise, the exercise can change to unlimited open training edged-weapon attacks as follows: you do not know which arm will launch the attack (right or left), what type of attack (straight, underhand, hook stab, or slash to the femoral artery, or variations of these), or the attack angle (straight or from an "off-angle") and height (high or low). The point is that you do not know what is coming.

You should train to defend against attacks and threats coming from all angles and heights. Attempt to incorporate specific techniques you have learned as best you can to defend an unanticipated attack. Importantly, most of these specific techniques should build on your defensive instincts. The technique may not always be performed correctly, but you will condition yourself to be proactive. Your ability to perform the optimum technique will improve over time as the techniques and reactions become more instinctive and ingrained. Defending against feints is also crucial to realistic training. You should combine all aspects of krav maga through retzev counterattacks to create explosive series of counterattacks using all parts of the body and weapons of opportunity. The following is a non-exclusive set of training drills to defend against armed attacks. Practice against both left- and right-handed attacks or threats with each type of weapon. You may also have your training partner incorporate strikes with his free arm or legs prior to and during the weapon's engagement.

Impact-Weapon Threat and Attack Pattern Drills

Work with a partner and a foam or rubber-type impact weapon to defend against the following non-exclusive list of mock attacks from all angles, including your training partner using both right- and left-handed grips:

1) The facsimile weapon is held in a threatening manner at different distances, grips, and postures. This should include hiding the weapon behind his leg or back
2) Horizontal strikes, both one-handed and two-handed variations, forehand, and backhand
3) X-strikes
4) Upside-down X-strikes
5) Low horizontal strikes
6) Over-the-top strikes

7) Thrusts, both one-handed and two-handed variations

8) Upside-down grip strikes

Edged-Weapon Attack Pattern Drills

Work with a partner and rubber edged weapon to defend against the following non-exclusive list of mock attacks from all angles, including your training partner using both right- and left-handed grips.

1) The facsimile weapon is held in a threatening manner at different distances, grips, and postures. This should include hiding the weapon behind his leg, back, or waistband. Variations include:

   a. Waiving the facsimile weapon in front of you

   b. Holding the facsimile weapon to your throat from the front

   c. Holding the facsimile weapon to your throat from the rear

   d. Holding the facsimile weapon to your back

   e. Pointing the facsimile weapon to your eye

   f. Other scenarios you can imagine

   g. Reacting with the appropriate defense before the weapon comes close to you

2) Over-the-top stabs, including one-handed and two-handed overhand variations

3) Overhead (icepick) stabs

4) Horizontal slashes

5) Hook stabs

6) X-pattern slashes

7) Upside-down X-slashes

8) Backhand stabs

9) Forward slashes and backslashes

10) Straight stabs to the neck, body, and groin

11) Underneath stabs to the groin and abdomen

12) Underneath (reverse grip) slashes up the center of the body

13) Low slashes to the groin and legs

14) Variations of these drills, when applicable, on the ground

Firearm Threats (Handgun, Submachine Gun (SMG), Rifle

Note: The handgun defenses should be practiced against both one- and two-handed grips.

1) Handgun in his waistband, front, side, and back (pre-deployment)

2) Handgun in his boot (pre-deployment)

3) Frontal threats including three heights—to the head, midsection, and groin

4) Frontal threats when you have a companion at your side

5) Frontal threats with the handgun concealed under a garment or in a coat pocket

6) Waiving the handgun in front of you

7) Side threats (three heights—to the head, midsection, and lower torso, including first-party hostage situations)

8) Rear threats (three heights—to the head, midsection, and small of the back, including first-party hostage situations)

9) Off-angle threats from all directions (three heights)

10) "Execution" defenses when defender is forced to kneel

11) Handgun with a push to front with the

   a. assailant's free hand
   b. barrel

12) Rifle/Submachine Gun (SMG) push to the front with the

   a. assailant's free hand
   b. barrel

13) Drill using defenses against a firearm in motion from all angles. The techniques remain the same, but the difficulty increases.

14) Variations of these drills, when applicable, on the ground

Defenses When Assailant is in Motion (Including Seated and Off-angle Attacks)

The assailant walks around the defender and attacks or threatens from all angles and directions as delineated in the previous drills:

1) Impact weapon
2) Edged weapon
3) Firearm

Partner Groundwork

1) Building on the above techniques, trainees work with one another on the ground. Usually, a weapon is most easily deployed when an opponent gains top position. The assailant sequesters a weapon or multiple weapons on his person. The assailant engages the defender in a mock fight on the ground. When opportune, the assailant should deploy the weapon and attempt to use it against the defender. The defender reacts using the appropriate technique as the situation dictates. In addition, if the defender notices during the mock confrontation a weapon or weapons, in the assailant's waistband, boot, or pocket—wherever the weapon might be—the defender must take appropriate action either confiscating the weapon or preventing the assailant from deploying it.

2) In another ground exercise, the assailant places facsimile weapons (impact and edged weapons along with firearms) strategically around the defender and grabs them for a quick interchange or attacks. These attacks should come rapid-fire. The goal is to have the defender react immediately without thinking—instinctively—the goal of krav maga.

Defending Against Two Armed Assailants

1) One assailant is armed with an impact weapon, the other with an edged weapon. Note: Defending against the impact weapon first is preferable to using the impact weapon against the edged weapon. However, circumstances—chiefly, proximity—may dictate defending the edged weapon first.

2) Two assailants armed with impact weapons. Note again, you must move to the deadside and debilitate, and control one of the assailants placing him in between you and the other assailant

3) Two assailants armed with edged weapons. Note again, you must move to the deadside and debilitate, and control one of the assailants placing him in between you and the other assailant

Special Training Scenarios

1) You are seated in a car and must use defenses against edged weapons and firearm threats through car windows. Note: If you intend a disarm attempt, it is advantageous to exit the vehicle before you engage, to afford you better mobility and an egress.

2) You are seated in a car and must use defenses against edged weapons and firearm threats from an assailant in either the passenger seat or rear seat. Note again, if you intend a disarm attempt, it is advantageous to exit the vehicle before you engage, to afford you better mobility and an egress.

3) You are seated in a simulated train or airplane seating from different angles, including seated, and other scenarios that come to mind.

4) You are seated or pinned to a wall (using all angles and directions).

Group Drills

Trainees form two lines and a student walks between the two and defends against weapon threats and attacks. Note: This is a good drill for unarmed scenario training as well.

Trainees work together in groups of four. One person is the designated defender. The other three students are called by number by the instructor or another trainee. Each trainee is armed with facsimile weapons, which could include an impact weapon, edged weapon, and firearm. The defender stands still while the three other students line up to the defender's left, center, right with the weapons in full view. One student is called or is otherwise designated to attack with a facsimile weapon. The goal is to practice immediate recognition of and reaction to many different threats and attack patterns from all angles and directions.

1) A variation of the above drill involves the defender standing still while the others walk around with the weapons behind their backs. Again, one trainee is called or is otherwise designated to attack with the facsimile weapon. If the defender sees the threat before it is deployed, he should perform the appropriate defense. The goal is to practice many different attacks from all angles and directions with different types of weapons and attack patterns.

2) The same drills can be repeated with the weapons shielded from the defender's view.

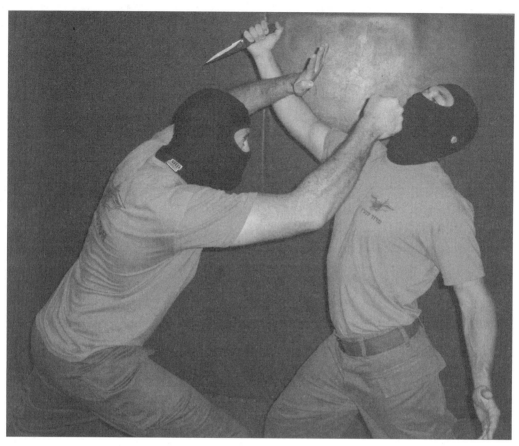

Sgt. Major (res.) Nir Maman (left in photo). Photo courtesy of Nir Maman.

Appendix
Vehicle Safety Tips, Road Rage, and Carjacking

Krav Maga Vehicle Safety Tips
---

1) Trust your instincts.
2) You are most vulnerable at

   a) Highway exit ramps.

   b) Intersections controlled by stoplights or signs

   c) Isolated garages or parking lots

   d) Park and ride lots for mass transportation

   e) Self-service gas stations or automobile washes

   f) Residential driveways

   g) ATMs

   h) Drive-through bank lanes

   i) Any other location where you must come to a stop

3) Avoid hitchhiking.
4) Do not make it easy for criminals to enter vehicle while you are driving. Lock your doors and avoid having open windows in a dangerous environment. Note: While bullets will penetrate automobile windows, law enforcement and security officials observe that criminals are less likely to shoot through a closed window.
5) Be wary in a parking lot of people asking questions or handing out flyers in close proximity to you.
6) If wary of a situation, you should approach your vehicle from the passenger side with your keys ready.
7) You should look into the rear seat to observe if another person might be present.
8) If you must a break a window, use your elbow covered with jacket or other useful tool.
9) Always look around before you egress from the vehicle.

10) If a suspicious person approaches you when your window is open, undo your seatbelt for a better reaction capability.

11) Let the assailant have the automobile if you are the only passenger or if everyone can safely exit the vehicle.

12) Safety techniques while driving to prevent carjacking:

   a) Do not tailgate; try to measure a safe distance by keeping the rear tires of the automobile in front of you in plain view.

   b) Drive in the center lane making it harder for carjackers to approach you.

13) If you are in an automobile and hit by another automobile:

   a) Survey the area before you get out. See if there are other vehicles or people around to observe the incident.

   b) Use your mirrors to observe who and what type of vehicle hit you.

   c) If you get of the vehicle, take your keys and vital possessions with you.

14) Park in well-lit locations near building entrances or walkways with heavy pedestrian traffic.

15) Avoid parking near dumpsters, wooded areas, large vehicles, or anything else that may afford a place for an assailant to hide.

16) Put valuables away in the trunk or hide them under something.

17) Open any automobile door twice to make sure of the possibility of escape.

Road Rage Incidents

Unfortunately, violent road rage conflict resulting from vehicular accidents or perceived slights is becoming all too common. Of course, the best way to handle road rage is to simply ignore the provocateur and drive away. However, sometimes you might be hemmed in and unable to escape. While you can remain in your vehicle buttoned down with your windows up and doors locked, your assailant can still assault you by shattering your window and following through with whatever ill intentions suit him. If you do choose to remain in your vehicle, you should unfasten your seatbelt in case you do have to quickly react.

If you are alone, the better plan is to egress from your vehicle and move to the far corner away from the aggressor. If you have passengers and the assailant becomes violent, obviously, you will react employing whatever skill set is necessary to interdict the assault. If the assailant threatens you and then moves toward his vehicle, you should quickly drive away, or if you cannot escape, you need to follow him to prevent his retrieving a possible weapon. A preemptive control hold might be necessary. As always, there are potential legal ramifications, including false imprisonment, if you by action or threat forcibly detain someone. You must be convinced that person has the intent and means to carry out his threat.

Carjacking When the Carjacker is Outside of Your Vehicle Brandishing a Firearm

Krav maga defenses against carjackers are the same principles you learned previously. There are some modifications if you must react when in your vehicle. A few essential scenarios begin to develop the krav maga practitioner's training approach.

For a basic overview, the key is having exited the vehicle is to react and disarm at the opportune time. While you can attempt disarms in the vehicle, you are in an inferior defensive position. In addition, you have probably practiced your weapons defenses primarily from a standing position. Obviously, it is best to react instinctively or as you have trained. Importantly, you cannot use lower body combatives or your full weight against the firearm. If you face multiple carjackers, decide if it is opportune to act as the others may also be armed and have multiple firearms aimed at you. Of course, as emphasized previously, no possession is worth risking your life over. Yet, if you have passengers in the car, especially children, you will have no choice but to react. It can be argued that reacting in the car allows you to drive away and drag a carjacker; however, the firearm will likely go off. If a passenger is sitting next to you, he or she may very well be put in the line of fire.

Defenses Against Carjacking Situations

According to the U.S. Bureau of Justice, firearms are used 45% of the time in carjackings. Of course, as emphasized previously, your life is not worth your automobile or its contents. You may have to react if you have a companion or child in the automobile who is in jeopardy of being kidnapped. The defenses against these types of scenarios are exactly the same as those previously covered depending on the scenario. You must exit the automobile to optimize the defenses. Timing, as always, is crucial to successfully neutralize the threat.

Carjacking Notes (according to Bureau of Justice Statistics 1993–2002)

- The majority (68%) of carjackings took place at night, particularly between 10:00 P.M. and 2:00 A.M.
- About 50% of all carjackings occurred in an open area such as on a public street or near public transportation.

- About 25% occurred in parking lots or garages near commercial places.
- About 75% occurred within five miles of the victim's home.
- 74% of all carjackings involved the use of a weapon. Firearms were used 45% of the time, knives accounted for 11%, and other weapons were used in 18% of the incidents.

Index

Biographies

Krav Maga Founder Imi Lichtenfeld

Krav maga founder Imi (Emerich) Lichtenfeld (1910-1998) was born in Budapest, Hungary and later resided in Bratislava, Slovakia. Prior to World War II, Imi faced increasing anti-Semitic violence. On the streets, Imi acquired hard-won experience and the crucial understanding of the differences between sport fighting and street fighting. Imi arrived in Israel after serving with great notoriety in the Czech Legion. Israel's early leaders immediately recognized Imi's fighting prowess and innovativeness. Imi began to train Israel's first fighting units the Palmach, Palyam, and Haganah in military close quarters combat. After retiring from the Israeli Defense Forces in 1964 as the chief hand-to-hand combat instructor, Imi established the Israeli Krav Maga Association (IKMA) in 1978 to promote krav maga throughout the world. Imi focused both on teaching professionals and adapting his system to provide ordinary civilians—men, women, and children—with solutions to avoid or end a violent encounter, or both.

Grandmaster Haim Gidon

Grandmaster Haim Gidon, 10th dan and Israel Krav Maga Association President, heads the Israeli krav maga (Gidon System) from the IKMA's main training center in Netanya, Israel. Haim was a member of krav maga founder Imi Lichtenfeld's first training class in the early 1960's. Along with Imi and other top instructors, Haim Gidon cofounded the IKMA. In 1995, Imi nominated Haim as the top authority to grant 1st dan krav maga black belt and up. Haim represented krav maga as the head of the system on the professional committee of Israel's National Sports Institute, Wingate. Grandmaster Gidon, whose professional expertise is in worldwide demand, has taught defensive tactics for the last three decades to Israel's security and military agencies. www.kravmagaisraeli.com.

Senior Instructor Yigal Arbiv

Yigal Arbiv (4th dan) is one of Grandmaster Haim Gidon's senior instructors. After serving in an elite paratroop unit as a weapons specialist, Yigal attended Wingate, Israel's national sports institute, an exclusive training academy for instructors and coaches to receive his krav maga coaching certification. Yigal is a security professional and krav maga instructor teaching in several schools in Israel. Yigal regularly travels abroad to teach law enforcement and civilians, having received special commendations from many American law enforcement agencies. Yigal sits on the IKMA's professional committee for krav maga technique development. info@kravmagaisraeli.com.

Senior Instructor Rick Blitstein

Rick Blitstein is one of a few handpicked individuals who traveled to Netanya, Israel in 1981 to complete an intensive krav maga instructor's course. Under the watchful eye of krav maga founder, Imi Lichtenfeld, Israeli experts taught Rick for the purpose of introducing krav maga in the United States. Imi and Rick formed very close bonds and spent much time training together in both Israel and the United States. For many of the past twenty years, Rick has worked in the field of private and corporate security, teaching and using krav maga in real-life situations. A member of the IKMA and recognized as a senior black belt instructor, Rick is committed to the proper expansion of the system in the United States and around the world. Rick sent his student David Kahn to train with the IKMA for instructor certification. Rick instructs in Miami and New York City. Rick also works as a professional fight coordinator for television and film, including ABC Television's *Charlie's Angels*.

Senior Instructor Alan Feldman

Alan Feldman is one the original martial arts instructors who received a scholarship to train in Israel in an intensive program to cultivate American instructors along with Rick Blitstein. Alan began teaching krav maga in the Philadelphia area in 1981. Alan is certified by the Israeli Ministry of Education and is one of the highest-ranking American instructors. Training directly under krav maga founder, Imi Lichtenfeld and his top ranked instructors, Alan has taught thousands of civilians in numerous schools, colleges, organizations, and agencies in addition to founding the first privately owned krav maga school in the United States. A member of the Israeli Krav Maga Association and recognized as a senior black belt instructor, over the years Alan was featured and recognized in numerous national publications. Alan teaches at the Israeli Krav Maga U.S. Training Center.

Instructor Abel Kahn

Abel Kahn began his krav maga training with David Kahn and completed his one-hundred-eighty-hour instructor training certification in Israel with Grandmaster Haim Gidon and Senior Instructor Yigal Arbiv. Abel is one of only a few Americans to complete Grandmaster Gidon's certification course in Israel and trains regularly in Israel. Abel is certified by the State of New Jersey Police Training Commission and has trained civilians and local, state, and federal law enforcement agencies in the United States. Abel has appeared in numerous publications including the *Daily News, Time Out, Absolute,* and in the book *Krav_Maga* and *Advanced Krav Maga*. Abel is responsible for the national rollout of Israeli krav maga in the United States in coordination with the Israeli Krav Maga Association.

Instructor/Photographer Rinaldo Rossi

Rinaldo Rossi began his krav maga training in 2001 and his advanced training with David Kahn 2006. Rinaldo completed his instructor certification with Grandmaster Haim Gidon and Senior Instructor Yigal Arbiv in both the United States and Israel. Rinaldo is one of only a few Americans to complete Grandmaster Gidon's certification course in Israel having tested in Israel for his advanced belt rankings. Rinaldo is responsible for the national rollout of Israeli krav maga in the United States with Don Melnick in coordination with the Israeli Krav Maga Association.

About the Author

David Kahn, IKMA United States Chief Instructor, received his advanced blackbelt teaching certifications from Grandmaster Haim Gidon and is the only American to sit on the IKMA Board of Directors. David has trained all branches of the U.S. military in addition to federal, state, and local law enforcement agencies. David is an instructor certified by the State of New Jersey Police Training Commission. Mainstream media regularly feature David including *Men's Fitness, GQ, USA Today, Los Angeles Times, Washington Post, New Yorker, Penthouse, Fitness, Marine Corps News, Armed Forces Network,* and *Military. com.* David previously authored the books *Krav Maga* and *Advanced Krav Maga* and produced the *Mastering Krav Maga* DVD series. David and his partners operate several Israeli Krav Maga Training Centers. For more information contact info@israelikrav.com or

Israeli Krav Maga U.S. Main Training Center
860 Route 206
Bordentown, New Jersey, 08505
(609) 585-MAGA
www.israelikrav.com

Israeli Krav Maga Association (Gidon System)
POB 1103
Netanya, Israel
www.kravmagaisraeli.com

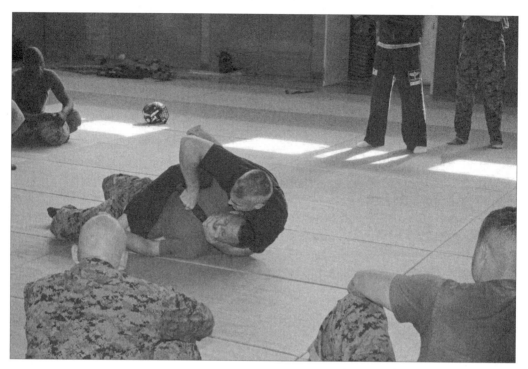

Training U.S. Marines. Photo courtesy of USMC Combat Camera.

Resources

For protective equipment and other supplies:

Asian World of Martial Arts
9400 Ashton Road
Philadelphia, PA. 1911 (800) 345-2962
www.awma.com

BLUEGUNS®
Ring's Manufacturing
99 East Drive, Melbourne, FL 32904
(321) 951-0407
www.blueguns.com

Authentic Israel Army Surplus
U.S. Local Phone: (718) 701-3955
Toll Free Number: (888) 293-1421
Israel (972) 3-6204612; Fax: (972) 9-8859661
P.O.B 31006, Tel Aviv, 61310, Israel
www.israelmilitary.com

To read more about krav maga and its history:

The Israel Defense Forces
Homepage: www.idf.il

The Israeli Special Forces
Homepage: www.isayeret.com

Israeli Special Forces Krav Maga
Homepage: www.ct707.com

Israeli Krav Maga Association
Homepage: www.israelikrav.com and www.kravmagaisraeli.com

DVDS FROM YMAA

more products available from …

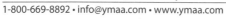

YMAA Publication Center, Inc. 楊氏東方文化出版中心

1-800-669-8892 • info@ymaa.com • www.ymaa.com

BOOKS FROM YMAA

more products available from . . .

YMAA Publication Center, Inc. 楊氏東方文化出版中心

YMAA
PUBLICATION CENTER

1-800-669-8892 • info@ymaa.com • www.ymaa.com